HOW TO SURVIVE

A BRAZILIAN BETRAYAL

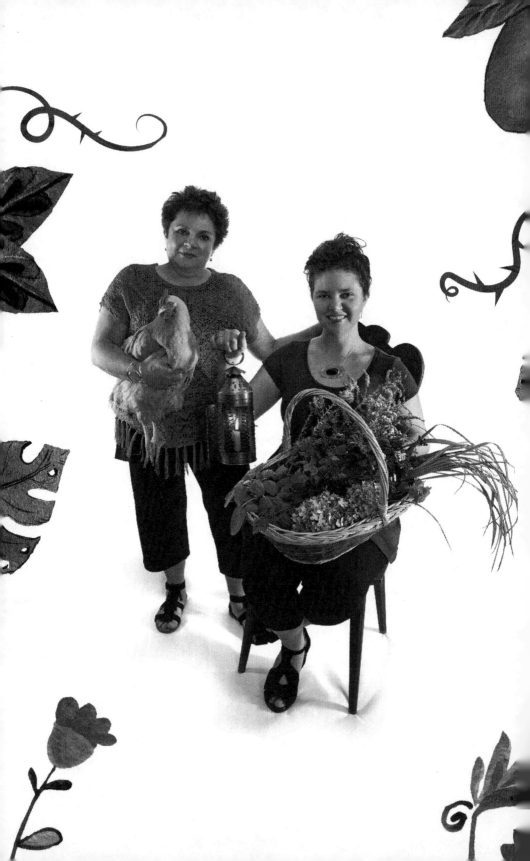

HOW TO SURVIVE A BRAZILIAN BETRAYAL

❀A MOTHER/DAUGHTER MEMOIR❀

Velya Jancz-Urban

&

Ehris Urban

Kelsey,
Don't be
afraid of
the wild
in you.
♡Ehris

Kelsey,
There is no
growth
without change...
With thanks,
Velya

GREEN WRITERS PRESS } *Brattleboro, Vermont*

Printed in the United States

10 9 8 7 6 5 4 3 2 1

Green Writers Press is a Vermont-based publisher whose mission is to spread a message of hope and renewal through the words and images we publish. Throughout we will adhere to our commitment to preserving and protecting the natural resources of the earth. To that end, a percentage of our proceeds will be donated to environmental activist groups and The Southern Poverty Law Foundation. Green Writers Press gratefully acknowledges support from individual donors, friends, and readers to help support the environment and our publishing initiative. Green Place Books curates books that tell literary and compelling stories with a focus on writing about place—these books are more personal stories/memoir and biographies.

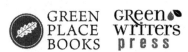

GREEN PLACE BOOKS   GREEN WRITERS PRESS

Giving Voice to Writers & Artists Who Will Make the World a Better Place
Green Writers Press | Brattleboro, Vermont
www.greenwriterspress.com

ISBN: 978-1-7327434-3-4

COVER DESIGN BY ASHA HOSSAIN DESIGN, LLC
BOOK DESIGN BY RACHAEL PERETIC
AUTHOR PHOTOS BY LORA KARAM PHOTOGRAPHY

PRINTED ON PAPER WITH PULP THAT COMES FROM FSC-CERTIFIED FORESTS, MANAGED FORESTS THAT GUARANTEE RESPONSIBLE ENVIRONMENTAL, SOCIAL, AND ECONOMIC PRACTICES. ALL WOOD PRODUCT COMPONENTS USED IN BLACK & WHITE OR STANDARD COLOR PAPERBACK BOOKS, UTILIZING EITHER CREAM OR WHITE BOOKBLOCK PAPER, THAT ARE SUSTAINABLE FORESTRY INITIATIVE® (SFI®) CERTIFIED SOURCING.

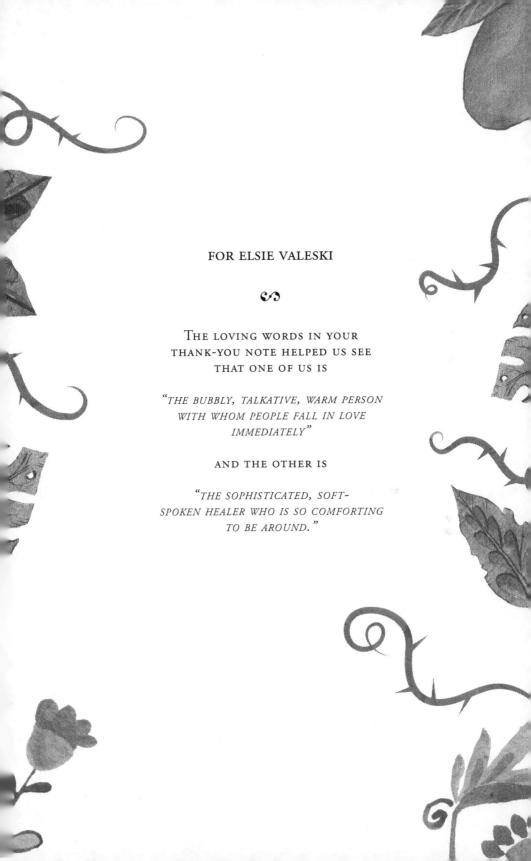

FOR ELSIE VALESKI

❧

THE LOVING WORDS IN YOUR
THANK-YOU NOTE HELPED US SEE
THAT ONE OF US IS

*"THE BUBBLY, TALKATIVE, WARM PERSON
WITH WHOM PEOPLE FALL IN LOVE
IMMEDIATELY"*

AND THE OTHER IS

*"THE SOPHISTICATED, SOFT-
SPOKEN HEALER WHO IS SO COMFORTING
TO BE AROUND."*

PROLOGUE
ℰↄ

Ehris

I was 16 when I realized it was all a sham.

"Who are we supposed to trust?" my mom asked when we got back in the car. "Jose or Guilherme?"

"I don't know," I said from the back seat, glancing up at Guilherme and Zoe's apartment building. "We've known Jose for like eleven years. We just randomly met this guy."

My mom, sweaty as usual from the Brazilian heat, said, "Ehris, back up for a sec. Can you translate *exactly* what Guilherme just told us again, so we're not getting screwed up by the Portuguese?"

"Jose told Guilherme that we're rich, entitled Americans who wanted to buy his farm and move to Ponte Nova to profit off cheap Brazilian labor. According to Guilherme, Jose lied to us about the price of the farm and stole all that extra money we sent him. Plus, he never gave Guilherme the final payment on the farm."

"So why did Guilherme suddenly tell us all this stuff tonight?" my mom asked.

"He said that when he and Zoe got to know us and realized we were *gente boa*, they felt terrible about what they'd done, and had to tell us the truth."

My dad was creepily staring out the windshield. The streetlights from the town square illuminated the lady selling homemade Nutella-gruyère waffle cones.

"This *would* explain why Jose's not answering our phone calls," my mom deduced.

My dad broke his silence, declaring, "We have to decide who's telling the truth."

When I closed my eyes and leaned back into the head-rest, highlights of Jose flashed through my mind. The time he and I were strapped into the front car of the Boulder Dash roller coaster at Lake Compounce, and he screamed even louder than I did. I was wearing a pink eyelet dress the day Jose bought a huge bucket loader, and he convinced me to be the first one to test drive it around his farm. A bunch of random Brazilian guys hung off the machine and shouted instructions at me in Portuguese, but I couldn't hear what they were saying. When I swung the bucket around, I just missed shattering his clay tile roof. "Ehriszinha," Jose laughed, "I no give you license!" The time we stuffed Jose into my dad's blue snowsuit when we all went skiing at Mohawk. When I raised the chairlift's safety bar at the top of the mountain, Jose's hood somehow got snagged. "Jeem! Jeem!" he howled to my dad. "Help! You no believe!" It all happened so fast that even the chairlift operator couldn't stop laughing as Jose scrambled to rip the furry hood off the snowsuit, dangled for just a second, then face-planted into the snow.

My heart couldn't believe it when I said, "I think we should trust Guilherme."

A *knock-knock* on my window spooked me. "Who the heck is that?" my mom asked as she whipped around.

"It's Guilherme," I said, rolling down my window.

"*Oi*, Ehriszinha," he greeted. "I saw your car from the apartment window. Zoe and I were talking after you left, and there's one more thing you have to know." I translated what Guilherme had said so far for my parents. He continued, "Jose left me a voicemail last week. I didn't want to scare you, but I think you have to hear this."

"*Ta bom, o que foi?*" (Okay, what is it?) I asked, opening the car door so Guilherme could sit next to me.

As Guilherme put his phone on speaker, Jose's familiar voice came on, but with an edge I'd never heard before. "*Você ja me perguntou muitas vezes sobre o pagamento da fazenda. Você não vai receber seu dinheiro. Lembre-se de que eu sei aonde você e sua mulher moram.*"

I translated the message without really digesting it: "You've asked me too many times about the farm payment. You're not getting your money. Remember, I know where you and your wife live."

"Jesus fucking Christ," my dad slowly muttered.

Guilherme added gravely, "I was talking to my friend at the bakery yesterday, and he told me he heard a rumor Jose killed a guy."

"He *killed* a guy?" my mom screeched after I translated.

Guilherme made purposeful eye contact with my dad and said carefully, "Ehris, tell your father that I think your family could be in danger."

My dad's hands clenched the steering wheel. "We have to get out of this fucking country."

PART ONE

This is part of what a family is about, not just love. It's knowing that your family will be there watching out for you. Nothing else will give you that. Not money, not fame, not work.

—MITCH ALBOM,
Tuesdays with Morrie

CHAPTER ONE

Velya

When Ehris and Mic were little, I had a framed index card on my desk. On the card was a typed quotation from the film *National Velvet*, which is not a kiddy horse tale or a simple movie about a horse-crazy tween. The film is about family—and about will and desire. It's about dreams—big and small, wise and foolish, realized and impossible, and about the way dreams change those who are lucky (or brave) enough to dream them.

Much of what I learned about being a mother came from *National Velvet*'s Araminty Brown, Velvet's very wise mother. It's the attic scene—one of the sweetest scenes ever filmed—that always makes the tears slide from my eyes. Mrs. Brown takes out the 100 gold sovereign coins she won for swimming the English Channel as a teenager, and gives them to Velvet to use as the entry fee for the Grand National horse race. There were many, many times the family could have used that money, but Mrs. Brown was saving it for a dream as big as her own once was. She tells Velvet, "I too believe that everyone should have a chance at a breathtaking piece of folly once in his life."

It was at least 20 years ago, long before Google and the internet, that I played that attic scene on our VCR and rewound the VHS tape over and over again, scribbling the lines on a yellow legal pad, until I had the text for my index card. I still know them by heart:

"Things come suitable to the time, Velvet. Enjoy each thing, forget it, and go on to the next. There's a time for everything. A time for having a horse in the Grand National, being in love, having children. Yes, even for dying. All in proper order at the proper time."

I used to be one of those people who thought they had everything figured out, and *because* I had everything figured out, nothing could go wrong. I contributed to a 401K, had cans of SPAM on hand in case the power went out, made sure there were ice scrapers in all the cars, was repentant when I lit a "fancy" candle that I "didn't want to waste," kept 26 years of monthly receipts from Northeast Utilities and SNET, never opened more than one jar of jelly at the same time, and saved the recipe for the hardtack I made for my students in 1982 when I tried (unsuccessfully) to liven up *The Red Badge of Courage*.

If our "breathtaking piece of folly" had worked out the way we planned, I would still be arranging the clothes in my closet in ROYGBIV order, missing out on dreams I never even knew I had.

CHAPTER TWO

Ehris

My mom is a charismatic weirdo. People gravitate to her for some reason. After one of her recent presentations of *The Not-So-Good Life of the Colonial Goodwife*, an older guy rushed up to the podium and told her about his first disastrous condom-buying experience. When she shared the guy's entire story with me in the car, I was like, "Eww! What did that have to do with a talk about colonial women? Why do people tell you this stuff?"

When I go into the Woodbury Post Office, it's a quick trip. There are no personal conversations. I say, "Can I mail this?" They say yes, I pay, and I leave. Yesterday, I waited in the car while my mom ran in to buy stamps. She was only gone four minutes. *Four* minutes. As she buckled her seat-belt, she prattled, "So, Dino can only eat peanuts when he's at work. His son has a peanut allergy. The kid has an EpiPen, and has had to inject himself a few times. You know how Mic told us that Corin is pregnant? I just told her that I had no idea, because I'm so short, I can't see over the counter. She was cracking up. I stood on tippy-toes to see her, and man, Ehris, she's going to have that baby any day!"

At least once a week, someone tells my mom she looks just like Liza Minnelli or Judy Garland. Last month, we were in an antique store (again), looking for a pierced tin lantern (again). The shop owner scampered over to my mom and announced, "Liza, I'm going to serenade you!" With that, she scurried over to the piano in the middle of the store, lifted the keyboard cover, and energetically belted a throaty rendition of "New York, New York."

Then there was the car wash. As I fed quarters into the self-serve vacuum, my mom wandered over to the dumpster. The car was so full of dried mugwort leaves and flowers that I had to put more quarters in. When the vacuum buzzed off the second time, she *still* wasn't back. It wasn't until I put the floormats, my yoga mat, and the library books back in the car that she finally reappeared, carrying a metal sign.

"Why do you have a Jack Daniel's Tennessee Honey whiskey sign?" I asked, rolling my eyes. "You don't even drink!"

"Okay, so, the bee on the sign wearing the helmet caught my eye. And then, the car wash guy invited me into his back room to show me all the loot that people just dump here. Oh, my god, Ehris, he had like seventy-five phone chargers, and enough cable wire to open a phone company. He showed me this humongous bag of clothes from Marshall's that still had price tags on them, and they pull $400 a month of jewelry out of the vacuum! I don't want the sign, but he made me take it, and I felt bad saying no."

This is life with my mom. People just like being around her. Everyone talks about her enthusiasm and energy. With fascination, people ask, "What it's like to have a mom like her?" It's like simultaneously wanting to shove a sock in her mouth, while admiring her gregariousness. My mom is nothing like me, and everything like me. She's the life of the party, and I don't even want to be *at* the party. But we're both creative, open-minded, offbeat, and resilient.

Velya

Just because Ehris doesn't say much, it doesn't mean people don't notice her. It's actually the quiet ones who often draw the most attention.

You so *don't get her*, I'd think at every single parent-teacher conference at Burnham Elementary School. Eventually, Jim and I gave up trying to explain, "No, she isn't shy; she's observant."

I looked out the kitchen window the other day, and studied Ehris as she used her hive tool to pry open the lid from one of her beehives. She removed the queen cage from the wooden box of 10,000 bees. And then, without wearing gloves, a baggy bee suit, or a veil, she introduced them to the hive. They quietly buzzed around her, and, like a flower, she let the bees come to her.

In Brazil, I watched Jim watch Ehris as she coaxed our obstinate mule, Jambi, over to the corral fence. Nobody, and I mean *nobody*, could even get close to this pigheaded mule. Jim didn't stop her when she climbed the fence and hoisted herself, bareback, onto dusty Jambi. I've always liked photos that are taken from behind, and the image I hold of the two of them loping through a field of *brachiaria* typifies Ehris's gift. *That's our girl*, I thought with pride. In a world of houseplants that become rootbound in pots, Ehris is a wildflower blooming in a meadow.

Never underestimate a quiet person. They are some of the most perceptive and absorbent people of all. Ehris is the eye of the hurricane. When a storm whirls and twirls, the calm power that drives it dwells at the very center.

CHAPTER THREE

Ehris

If you have an unusual name, you understand that this is both a blessing and a curse. People get kind of thrown off when they hear your name, and it usually takes them some time before they get used to pronouncing it. As people wonder about the roots of your name, it becomes a topic of conversation.

My name, which is sort of pronounced like "heiress," comes from my maternal grandmother's maiden name, which is Ehrismann. A few times a year, I get a piece of mail addressed to Mr. Chris Urban. Last month, someone thought my name was "Ursula." I spent eight weeks of swimming lessons being called "Iris." My favorite was the time I won a photo contest and the *Litchfield County Times* captioned me as "Elvis Urban."

My mom's name, Velya, is pronounced "Vealia," and comes from the Viennese *Merry Widow* operetta. "Vilja" was the Witch of the Woods. When my brother, Mic, and I learned this, he was like, "Witch of the woods! Yo, Nazey got that one right!" My mom says that during her two years at East Ridge Junior High ("the worst two years of my life"), she constantly heard, "Velya, I wanna feel ya!" People from her old life call her "Veal."

Nazey is my maternal grandmother. Her real name, Neysa (pronounced Nay-suh), comes from a famous illustrator in the 1920s, Neysa McMein (who was actually born Marjorie, but discarded the old-fashioned name and christened herself Neysa after a racehorse she admired). Mic and I never called her Grandma. To us, she was Nazey.

While I've never found a keychain or mug with my name on it, having an unusual name has encouraged me to march to the beat of my own drum.

It was my great-grandmother, Ann, who started the tradition of unusual names. She was a flapper, knew how to drive, and carefully chose a unique name for her daughter, Neysa. Ann abandoned ten-year-old Neysa along with her five-year-old brother, Chuck, in 1936. Nobody knows the reason she left, but she later remarried and had two more kids. Just as a single mold spore pollutes a slice of bread and eventually covers the entire loaf in a contaminated green blanket, my great-grandmother Ann's action affected everyone in my family.

I feel like I've lived two separate lives. Even though I'm only 25, lifetime number one seems so long ago. Sometimes I wonder, *was that even me?* My memories are sprinkled with mental amnesia. It's a weird feeling to not know how much you don't remember. I guess my brain is protecting me from stuff I don't want to think about.

It's kind of like something else that happens once in a while. Sometimes, my mom, dad, or I will be looking for something we used to have when we lived in the Bridgewater house. Suddenly, we'll realize that we haven't seen that thing in over nine years, and it's just one of the many things that have disappeared. Maybe it fell off the cargo container into the Atlantic Ocean, or something. It happened just the other day, when I asked, "Whatever happened to that jar of corn-on-the-cob holders?" It's always something we can live without. But it's something that played a role in my first life—just like my grandparents.

Velya

There's this thing I do. Every time I watch a Turner Classic Movie on TV, I automatically calculate how old my mother, Neysa, would have been when she saw the original film in a theater. I picture her in an above-the-knee cotton dress with a Peter Pan collar, kind of like the ones Darla, the coquettish love interest of Alfalfa, wore in *The Little Rascals* comedies. I see her alone in the dark with a five-cent box of Raisinets in one of those grand old theaters in Jersey City. The Stanley Theater opened in 1928, and had 4,300 seats and two crystal chandeliers—one of which was illuminated by 144 bulbs reflecting onto 4,500 hanging crystal teardrops. When King Kong fought that airplane on top of the Empire State Building, my mother would have been seven years old. When lightning struck a kite that sent electricity through the Bride of Frankenstein, she was nine. When Mr. Smith went to Washington and Dorothy skipped down the yellow brick road, she had just turned 13. I see her there in the Stanley, the closest she would get to a palatial setting, escorted to her velvet seat by a uniformed usher and settling in for a double feature plus cartoon. And for as long as it takes to play out this scenario in my mind, my mother is still a little

Depression-era girl, blissfully unaware that she will one day die in a Connecticut nursing home.

In the year following my mother's death, I literally and metaphorically never went in reverse. The metaphoric part involved my heart, which I never allowed to think about the past. I forced my brain to become one of those revolving automated racks at a dry cleaner. Any thought that involved my mother got put back on the rack, and I mentally pushed the button to make it go away.

One memory *did* sneak through when I let myself dwell too long in one of my "how old was my mother when this movie was released" reveries. Along with most of the population, my mother's family was incredibly poor during the Great Depression. New clothes were a rarity for her, so you can imagine her delight when a friendly man cozied up next to her in a plush movie theater seat at the Stanley and admired her pretty dress.

"My, that's a lovely new dress you're wearing," he complimented her.

My mother, initially flattered, wondered how the man knew her dress was new as he ran his hand up and down her chest to feel its material.

"I'll tell you what," he offered. "I'll give you a nickel for a box of candy if you promise to come right back and sit next to me," he smiled, patting the seat she was in.

My mother agreed. She took his nickel, danced up the carpeted aisle to the three-story lobby, bought a box of Nonpareils (those dark chocolate discs sprinkled with small white candy balls), and happily ensconced herself in one of the 4,300 seats of the Stanley, as far away as she could possibly get from the pervert.

She loved telling that story, and on the very rare occasions when she ate candy, they were always Nonpareils—or Non-parallels, as my brother, Jordan, and I called them.

The literal part of never going in reverse, that year after my mother's death, involved my car. It was a 1991 black Mercedes 560 SEL with heated reclining front and back seats, rear-seat foot rests, and an incredible mirror finish. It was the kind of car that men always commented upon when I loaded the trunk with groceries or pumped gas. The fit and finish left no doubt that the absolute best of every material had gone into the car's construction. Jim had bought it (used) for its battering-ram-solid sense of security, but it always felt like a chauffeur should have been behind the wheel, with a diplomat in the back seat and Jimmy Hoffa in the trunk.

One day, in that year of grief and repressed memories, the big black Benz just stopped going in reverse. The mechanic's estimate to have the car repaired was sky-high.

"I'll just keep driving it the way it is," I stubbornly told Jim. After 32 years of marriage, he had become an expert at "interpreting Velya." He had no trouble with the translation: "I deserve to be punished—but I don't want anyone else to do it for me. I have to punish myself."

"Wifely, you know how many times we tried to help your mother, but she wouldn't help herself. No one blames you," Jim assured me.

That doesn't matter, I thought. *Not when you blame yourself.*

And so, for a year, I never went in reverse. There were no more trips down Memory Lane because that would have required going backward. I came to a lot of intersections, and couldn't just back up. So I learned to focus on the front windshield and not the rearview mirror. Life is a constant motion forward, and driving is about constant adjustments. You always have to pay attention.

I developed a routine, albeit a weird one. I would take aimless drives and play Jim Brickman's *Destiny* cassette tape. Years before, I had bought the tape at Goodwill for 50 cents. One of the tracks was a recording of "The Rainbow Connection." Everyone knows this song—it's the one Kermit sings in that swamp while plucking his banjo at the beginning of *The Muppet Movie*. In his intro to the song, Jim Brickman talks about possibilities, hopes, dreams, wishes, and inspiration, and how you never really know what's coming next in your life. I would let the song play, and then rewind it and play it over, and over, and over again.

Even as this was all happening, I knew I was acting nutty. Of course, I was grieving, but I was also thinking. I knew that all of the puzzle pieces from my old life could never fit back into the puzzle. I had to give myself permission to let go of those extra pieces and move on. It's all about the three Cs: choices, chances, change.

CHAPTER FOUR

Velya

My mother taught me the art of walking on eggshells. Jordan, my mother, and I stepped gingerly around my father's personality disorder, but when you're a kid, you never really know what goes on in other people's houses. Didn't all mothers slip a tranquilizer in the after-dinner coffee of their husbands? She'd wink at Jordan and me and say, "Lucrezia's paying a little visit tonight," referencing Lucrezia Borgia, who, it was rumored, was in possession of a hollow ring she frequently used to poison drinks.

We had a kooky Filipino doctor, the closest thing my mother had to a friend. She wore polyester tank tops and scuffed around in slippers. Her office was in the basement of her house, and my mother called her Becky. At our first appointment, her husky ten-year-old son answered the door in white brief underwear and ushered us into the waiting room, which was decorated with brightly colored wooden masks. After every office visit, she'd invite us upstairs for tea, served in her mother's collection of translucent bone china tea cups. She couldn't say the letter V, and therefore evaporate became *ebaporate*, Velya become *Belya*, and varicose veins were *baricose beins*.

My mother and Becky were in cahoots. She prescribed Librax for my father, convincing him it would help his hiatal hernia. In reality, Librax helped *us*. Since it was an anti-anxiety medication, it tranquilized my father. He took it on a daily basis.

On days when one pill didn't do the trick and my mother sensed impending doom, he got a second dose in his coffee. My mother was quite adept at twisting open the pale green capsule and dumping the contents in his coffee cup while he sat in the dining room waiting for dessert: Entenmann's Crumb Coffee Cake and instant coffee with sedatives and milk. "We never lie to Daddy, but we don't have to tell him everything, either," became her mantra.

What did it say about my family that some of my strongest memories were of my mother calling my father names behind his back? She said he was emotionally immature, always had to be the center of attention, liked to hurt people with his words, and sought admiration by devaluing others.

When Ehris and Mic were quite little, not much more than chubby-fingered toddlers, I found a pale blue china tea set, complete with tea pot, cups, saucers, and adorable little plates, at a cluttered antique store. Its enameling and gilding were in mint condition. I had no intention of preserving this delicate set in a glass-front china cabinet like an off-limits museum piece. I bought it for our kids to use at tea parties.

Over the years, many, many chocolate chip cookies graced the fragile plates. Milk poured from the spouted teapot to the dainty teacups with gilt handles so small, even Jim's pinkie couldn't fit through the opening. Our kids knew this tea set was very special, yet they also knew if something broke, it wouldn't be the end of the world. I've always believed that kids will rise to the occasion if given the opportunity, which is why we took Ehris and Mic to good restaurants, Broadway plays, hospital rooms, concerts, funerals, dinner theaters, and meetings with lawyers and accountants. We included them in all family decisions.

Our cedar chest dress-up box held exquisite evening gowns, white satin gloves that practically reached the armpits of a four-year-old, embroidered kimonos with silk frog closures, clip-on dangly rhinestone earrings, and purple sequined high heels that would make even Carrie Bradshaw and Imelda Marcos drool. The kids always tea-partied in their dress-up finery, yet nothing was ever broken—not even a chip appeared on any of the intricate floral-patterned pieces. None of this seemed very remarkable to me, but my mother continually marveled at what a wonderful idea it was to entrust the fragile tea set to the kids.

Recently, a forgotten childhood memory popped vividly into my mind, and I suddenly understood my mother's praise. My parents had a set of gaudy cocktail glasses given to them by the best man at their wedding. Perhaps the amber long-stemmed glasses had been fashionable in 1949, the year they married. I don't ever remember us using them. They were high up on the forbidden shelf in the pantry, along with some cut-glass bowls. On the rare times my mother took the bowls down and flicked them with her finger, they would ring, signifying they were real cut glass.

I don't know why I was holding one of the amber glasses in the dining room that night, but I do know I was very little. I don't remember dropping it, or the way the amber glass must have shattered as it hit the linoleum floor—the same earth-tone, fake brick pattern that everyone in Connecticut seemed to have in the 1960s. But I do remember my father. He exploded with animal rage, his eyes a maniacal frenzy, and charged to the living room. He returned holding my Tiny Tears doll, with her white romper and rock-a-bye eyes. Standing right in front of me, with the veins bulging out of his neck, he tore her head off. He screamed, "How does it feel to see me break something that belongs to you?"

How did it feel, Dad? It felt like the amber cocktail glass was more important than I was.

Deep down, was that why I bought the tea set? Did I want my children to understand that things can always be replaced, but broken feelings can't be mended? That there should never be a forbidden shelf in your home—or in your heart?

I never saw my mother touch those glasses again.

Ehris

When I was little, I never realized how messed up my grandparents were. I don't know how I didn't notice, but I guess my grandfather was tranquilized most of the time, so maybe that's why.

"Hey, Ehris, wanna hear a story about life with Nazey and Grandpa?" Uncle Jordan once asked.

"Sure," I said.

"You know those blue and white delft shot glasses that were on the shelf in their pantry?"

"Yeah, I remember they had little windmills on them," I said.

"When I would come home from junior high, Nazey would let me lie on the couch and watch *Lost in Space*. Then she would give me one of those shot glasses, filled to the brim with Vandermint."

"Wait. Isn't that the chocolate mint liqueur stuff?" I asked.

"Yeah. I would sip it, and then drink a few more shots. She told me it would 'take the edge off.'"

"Weren't you like eleven?"

"Yup," Uncle Jordan said crisply. "And your mom was around thirteen. She never got the Vandermint treatment because she never rocked the boat."

"I don't get it. Why did you need to 'take the edge off' when you were eleven?"

"I guess it made it easier for her if Grandpa and I were both medicated," he explained. "Then there wouldn't be any drama between us when he came home from work."

"But my mom always said you were such a nice little kid," I responded.

"I was." He shrugged. "But it seemed like no matter what I did, in his eyes, it was always wrong. I guess if I was kind of drunk, and he was kind of tranquilized, dinnertime was bearable."

"Wow. I'm surprised you two were able to pass the tuna noodle casserole around the table!"

Of course, giving Vandermint to your pre-teen and drugging your husband with Librax aren't the best ways to deal with problems, but Nazey never dealt with issues directly. On her nightstand, she had self-help books from the 1960s like *I'm OK, You're OK* and *Games People Play*, which analyzed how to deal with difficult people. The books' themes addressed the fact that nobody can affect you but you, and you control your destiny. She read all this stuff, but never incorporated any of it into her life. She was wise, but not really.

Nazey would type insightful, cryptic messages on blank index cards with her Royal typewriter and tape them to the fridge, bathroom mirrors, and bookshelves. Most of them were intended for my grandfather, who was clueless. He never made the connection between the "feel-good hippie crap" and improving his personal relationships. The cards said things like:

Criticize the act, not the child.

Walk away from destructive people.

You are the master of the unspoken word; once it leaves your lips, you are its slave forever.

More marriages are broken due to bad manners than to infidelity.

There is no growth without change.

"Grandpa is emotionally immature," Nazey would share with me when I was in elementary school, way too young to be hearing this stuff. "He always plays the *see what you made me do* and the *yes, but* game," she'd confide, quoting from her books. But then she'd say something ridiculous, like, "Kids, especially sons, should always have a little bit of fear around their fathers."

In different ways, my grandparents were equally baffling. Nazey spent an absurd amount of her life plotting ways to hide things from my grandfather—things she was convinced would "set him off." Not to excuse him, because he *was* unpredictably explosive, but it was like the "chicken or the egg" debate. Did she lie to him because he was like volatile and unstable nitroglycerin, or had he become this way because she was always doing things behind his back?

"Here's the money for the things I put on your credit card when we went to Kohl's the other day," Nazey would say, handing my mom some tightly folded ten dollar bills. They were always ten dollar bills, since they came from the allowance my grandfather put on her dresser each week. "Grandpa doesn't care what I buy, but now I don't have to explain anything to him," she'd say illogically, even though she had a job and her own credit cards.

"The next time you go see your naturopath, can you pick me up two bottles of those Garden of Life multivitamins?" she'd ask, passing my mom two empty vitamin bottles hidden in a small brown paper bag, so she'd know which ones to get, along with some cash. The brown paper bag prevented my grandfather from seeing what was inside when we left their house. "Grandpa doesn't care," she'd swear, "but he doesn't see why I can't just take the One A Day vitamins like he does."

For years, my mom smuggled Poise pads, and then Depends, into the house for her. "I don't want Grandpa to know about my bladder problem," she'd explain as we pulled the packages from the trunk while my grandfather was raking or food shopping.

As kids, my mom and Uncle Jordan were willing co-conspirators, because they had witnessed the consequences of my grandfather's fury. Something stupid, like not being able to find the special mallet and rope he used for the dreaded spring ritual of putting the dock in the lake, could lead to a week of silent treatment, threats of "selling the goddamn house," or promises of divorce.

My grandfather knew that these were the things that terrified all three of his victims the most. My mom became an emotional Geiger counter. Hyper-alert to radioactive shifts in my grandfather, she would employ all of her people-pleaser talents to defuse the black atmosphere of terror before it permeated the house. Since my mom couldn't fix something if she didn't know what was broken, to her, the silent treatments were the most poisonous punishments.

As soon as I was out of diapers, I was indoctrinated with the "three pees to a flush" rule when I used the bathroom at my grandparents' house. They took this very seriously. My grandfather was convinced that if they didn't baby the septic tank, the entire septic system would fail, and he wouldn't be allowed to replace it. When he was feeling extra paranoid, I think he extended the mandate to "11 pees to a flush." Even though I would hold my nose and try not to look at the brewing urine in the toilet bowl, fermenting into the color of Gulden's spicy brown mustard, it smelled worse than a Porta-Potty in July. The bathroom garbage can, full of used toilet paper since it wasn't allowed in the toilet, just added to the experience.

One day, when my mom was a teenager, she stood up from the toilet in the upstairs bathroom and her elbow hit the toilet paper holder. The toilet paper unrolled across the bathroom floor. To her horror, the wooden spindle flew off the holder and disappeared into the flushing toilet.

"Whatever we do, we can't tell Daddy about this," Nazey told my mom and Uncle Jordan. If toilet paper in the toilet was a crime, they could only imagine the wrath over a hexagonal wooden spindle lodged in the bowels of the pipes. "Here's what's going to happen," she instructed them. "You two can pee in this toilet, but not poop in it." This made no sense, but for over a year, they kept up this ruse.

Unbelievably, my grandfather never noticed that two kids were pooping in their bedroom bathroom. Finally, Nazey commanded, "Veal, I've had enough. Today's the day. Stick your hand down there and pull it out!" My mom gagged and retched, but plunged her hand down the toilet up to her shoulder (she exaggerates a lot), and eventually fished out the waterlogged wooden spindle. Nazey stuck the discolored spool through the toilet paper roll, and it's still in use in their upstairs bathroom.

For "his own good," my grandfather was kept in the dark about things like this incident, and the time my mom spilled a whole can of black enamel paint in the dryer while making a magic wand, and the baby skunk that nibbled leftover cat food by the side door every night.

Someone recently asked my mom, "What kind of woman was your mother? Was she kind?"

The question seemed to catch her off guard. "No, she wasn't kind, but she wasn't the opposite of kind, either," she answered.

"Nazey was secretive," I responded. "That's the first thing I thought of when you asked the question. It sounds bad, but that's how I think of her."

I know a lot of the secrets that Nazey, my mom, and Uncle Jordan kept from my grandfather. I know how much joy the three of them shared in the pantry every night as they peeked through the window, watching that adorable skunk grow up as it leisurely crunched Meow Mix. But I also know that when my grandfather found out about the skunk, he shot it with a B.B. gun as my mom sobbed, "No, no!" Before limping back to the woods, the skunk triumphantly blasted him, and the side of the house, with its anal scent glands. For years, every time it rained, the musk and the memory reactivated, ingraining the importance of secrecy in my mom.

My grandparents were two people destined to destroy each other, but neither of them would walk away.

CHAPTER FIVE

Velya

It always sounded ridiculous to me when my mother said she wanted to marry a man who went to work in a suit and tie. She met my father a few years after World War II ended. Courtesy of the G.I. bill, he was a night student at Pace College (which eventually became Pace University). She was willing to work full-time as a stunning receptionist in a prestigious New York City law firm, write and type his papers, and read required poetry and classics aloud to him on the weekends. He would provide the security and upward mobility she so strongly craved.

Abandoned by her mother when she was ten years old at the height of the Great Depression, my mother had adored the Andy Hardy movies of the early 1940s starring Mickey Rooney as Andy and Lewis Stone as the compassionate Judge Hardy, the gentle father who had man-to-man talks with Andy in his book-lined study. The movies were sappy comedies celebrating ordinary American life—snippets of an America untouched by the Depression or the war percolating in Europe. My mother knew that somewhere out there was a town just like the Hardy's fictional hometown of Carvel, Idaho, where nothing bad ever happened. A place where mothers did not desert their children, fathers were wise and strong, families held patriotic weenie roasts, and all the endings were happy ones. My father could give her Carvel, Idaho.

My mother's Carvel was Ridgefield. To be more specific, a waterfront house on tiny Rainbow Lake in Ridgefield, Connecticut, a suburban community in Fairfield County with the requisite 2.5 kids per family. In this affluent town, she raised two children, worked in the school system, and, in her own way, kept my father under control.

Secrecy became the pervasive fifth member of my family. My mother worked in the office of my elementary school, and later, in the guidance office of my high school. She was privy to all kinds of confidential information, like IQ scores, teen pregnancies, abortions, kids in rehab, whose parents were divorcing or alcoholics, and who had gone into the boys' bathroom at Ridgebury Elementary School and stuck a toothpick all the way up his penis. Perversely, she shared all of this with us, but only after extracting our solemn oaths of silence.

Why did she do this? I think it had something to do with being abandoned as a child. She always told us that each year, as she blew out the candles on her birthday cake, she wished, "I hope Momma comes home. I hope Momma comes home." One year, she told us she wised up and actually said to herself, "You dope, Momma's never coming home." She claimed the love she felt from her father and her mother's four sisters made up for her mother's absence. Unbelievably, I bought this line until very recently, when Jordan pointed out, "Veal, come on, think about it. Nobody could ever be okay with their mother deserting them."

My mother always told us that there was never any shouting or yelling between her parents. She remembers her father calling for a taxi and her mother getting in and leaving. Maybe the most painful goodbyes are the ones that are never said—and never explained. My mother's secrecy and attempts to prove the superiority of her own little nuclear family may have masked her fear of abandonment.

To my mother, compared to where she came from, Ridgefield was a jewel, as was the house—"a jewel within a jewel," she extolled. In her mind, it was the nicest house in Ridgefield. From the flowering dogwood trees, cathedral ceiling, and lovely little upstairs dressing room, to the stone steps leading down to the wooden dock from which her children and grandchildren swam, sailed, and ice skated, my mother reveled in her New England utopia. To her, the house represented her legacy. Besides her college-educated children, it was the thing of which she was the most proud. Surrounded by acorn-heavy oak trees, early American fieldstone walls, and flagstone patios, the house was material proof of achieving the American Dream. It was a tangible reminder of how far she had come from Jersey City, the Great Depression, poverty, and abandonment.

I have mixed feelings about my mother. Of course, she allowed this to happen, but my father drove any friends and family she had out of her life. As little kids, we became her confidants. Children keep secrets. Children are loyal. It was an awkward dynamic, and she should have let her hair down with girlfriends and used them as sounding boards, instead. She should have set things straight with my father the very first time he pulled his shenanigans.

In 1949, when my parents were newlyweds, they lived in Jersey City, New Jersey. My mother was a receptionist at Alexander & Green, a white-shoe law firm in Manhattan. White-shoe meant it was owned by conservative WASP elites. My father saw a newspaper ad for whole hams on sale at Gristedes, and asked my mother to go buy one after work. In her high heels and pencil skirt, she click-clacked the 45 blocks from E 21st Street to E 66th Street, then held the 15-pound ham on her lap as she rode the train, and then the bus, home to their tiny apartment.

In old photos, my mother looked like a busty Olivia de Havilland. We often heard the story of how one day, during World War II, she was wearing a white blouse tucked into a navy skirt, cinched with a wide red-patent belt. A sailor passed her on the street, took off his sailor cap, pressed it to his heart, and said, "God Bless America."

I pictured her like that when I heard the ham story. She was typing one of my father's papers when he came home and spotted the ham. Like a kid having a tantrum, he jumped up and down on his fedora—which he had thrown on the floor—and roared that she had bought the wrong kind. "You can't even buy a goddamn ham!" he sneered. Instead of telling him where he could stick his stupid ham, she apologized and returned it the next day. That was when the walking on eggshells began.

CHAPTER SIX

Velya

I met Jim when I was 20 years old and we were both college students. It was early May, and I was sitting on a bench outside the student union, enjoying the glorious spring weather with my friends. Out of nowhere, a guy rushed up to me, handed me an open box of Wheat Thins, said they were left over from an oral presentation, and then literally ran away. Man, oh man, was I intrigued!

I saw the guy again two days later, at an outdoor party at one of the dorms. He walked up to me wearing a navy blue T-shirt, and I thought his chest looked just like a G.I. Joe doll's. You know the shape: two hard mounds with a valley down the center. He said his name was Jim, and that he already knew my name. Then he ran off again, saying he had to go to work. Interested? This went way beyond love at first sight. I knew I was going to marry this guy. I am absolutely serious. I knew it.

The next day there was a huge clambake sponsored by the fraternity this Jim guy belonged to. My friends were all on the beer line, and not being a beer or clam person, I was patiently standing on line for a hotdog. There, at the grill cooking and serving hotdogs, was Jim.

"Can I have a hotdog?" I asked.

He smiled. "For a kiss."

I got my hotdog, he got his kiss, and we were married four years later.

When Ehris and Mic first heard this story, they made gagging noises and rolled their eyes. This response was so unlike Jim, they couldn't possibly believe their father could have ever said anything this romantic. Long before Patrick Swayze responded "ditto" to Demi Moore when she told him she loved him in the 1990 film *Ghost*, Jim had been saying the same thing to me. He once gave me a cement mixer for a present! Then there was the time I spent hours getting ready for a New Year's Eve party, and thought I looked pretty snazzy in a green wraparound geometric-print dress. When I made my entrance, Jim looked at me for a second and said, "Wifely, you look blurry." I still don't know if this was supposed to have been a compliment.

On the flip side, Jim usually gets in bed first, and every night when I go into the bathroom to wash my face, my toothbrush sits next to the sink, topped with a minty white line of toothpaste—waiting for me like a love letter. It's there every morning, too. I find this gesture extremely tender.

Perhaps because my brother has been married three times, he tends to offer an extremely simple, yet complex piece of relationship advice: *accept love as it is offered.* In other words, it's important to recognize when someone is trying to show you love, even if it's not the way you want it. Jim and I have been married for 35 years. It would take a crowbar to pry the phrase "I love you" out of this man, yet I adore him. He is my man of action.

Eleven days before our wedding, Jim surprised me with 11 roses and a handwritten florist's card, which said: "One for each day left. I can't wait. I love you. I always will." He has never left the house without kissing me goodbye. This is how my husband offers his love. He rarely gives a compliment, but has always used three words: *us*, *we*, and *our* when he talks about our life. He protects what he loves and cherishes.

Jim and I chuckle when we think about the home improvements we made on our Bridgewater house, which was listed as a "handyman special." This was a house we bought after seven months of marriage.

We loved the fact that the house was located on four acres of land, because we knew a cookie-cutter subdivision wasn't for us. We didn't like the daycare idea, and always knew one of us would stay home once our kids were born, so we bought a house we could afford on one salary. We didn't have a lot of money, but we got such a kick out of planning our projects and designing additions. In the beginning, Jim used an upside-down plastic fuchsia bathroom garbage can as a sawhorse, and straightened out old bent nails in order to re-use them. Every Saturday morning, we would go out for breakfast, then spend $100 at the local lumberyard (it's amazing how far $100 went back then). Jim would work on the week's project until he ran out of supplies, while I graded papers and did lesson plans. Stylistically, it's not a good idea to repeat a word over and over. I was going to do some editing, but that's exactly how it's always been with Jim and me. Schmaltzy as it sounds, it's always been "we."

That time in our lives reminds me of my favorite romantic story. The legendary American actress Helen Hayes was married to the equally famous playwright,

Charles MacArthur. When she met Charles at a party in Manhattan, it was love at first sight when she looked across the room and saw him eating peanuts out of a paper bag. Later in the evening, he poured some salted peanuts into her hand and said, "I wish they were emeralds." Like any young couple, Helen and Charles struggled in the early years of their marriage. Many years later, on an important anniversary, Charles poured some emeralds into her lap and said, "I wish they were peanuts." I know exactly how he felt. If you don't get the story, it's hard to explain, but it's about struggling and building something together. It's about creating something with someone else, with the world stretched out before you.

It took years and years to finish our projects, and if you've ever owned a house, you know you're never really finished. I guess what I mean by *finished* is we reached the point when we were ready to start a family, and of course, that's when the house stopped being just a house.

It seems silly now, but I spent a lot of time wondering and worrying how I would know when the time was right to try and have a baby. I would see mothers kiss the tops of their babies' heads and wonder, *why do they have the urge to do that?* I clearly remember sitting in a mall and watching a mother wipe her kid's face with a wet washcloth she pulled from a Ziploc bag, wondering, *how did she even know to pack a wet washcloth?* It seemed like these women belonged to a mysterious club with a secret password. One night, when we were making love in our moonlit bedroom, Jim looked up at me and said, "Velya, I want to make babies with you." As simple as that. I knew it was time. The rest of my life was starting.

Jim and I waited seven years to try and have a baby, then had a hard time conceiving. After our first baby miscarried, we were devastated. I remember the purple turtleneck sweater I was wearing when we went in for the vaginal ultrasound. The doctor thought my uterus was a little large for the conception date, and suspected I might be carrying twins. Instead, there were no twins—just a dead baby.

I have absolutely no idea how we got from the darkened ultrasound room with the glowing monitor to the hospital room many floors below, where I had to have a blood test. Jim got me there. For years, the turtleneck sweater sat folded on a shelf in my closet, and there was always a feeling of avoidance about it. I never wore a turtleneck sweater again.

All of this happened just days before Christmas, and we had to wait five days before a D&C could be performed. Imagine what it's like to walk around trying to live with a dead baby inside you. I cried quietly as they wheeled me into the operating room, and was still crying when I woke up in the recovery room. I remember thinking, even through the anesthesia, that that was interesting. That was when I found out you don't have to be awake for your heart to be broken. An older nurse came over to me, put her arm around my shoulders, and said, "Just cry it out, honey." So many years later, those words still mean so much. I still remember, and will always remember, the date of that horrible ultrasound and the baby's due date. Every year, I think about how old the baby would be now. Jim made me whole again. I don't know who made Jim whole.

When Mic, and then two years later, Ehris, nursed, I would feel milk and love flowing from me. I had no idea about the intensity of love until I started caring for these new little creatures we had created together. As they brought us along with them on their journey, I finally learned the password.

CHAPTER SEVEN

Ehris

When I was a kid, Bridgewater was the only remaining "dry town" in Connecticut. It was illegal to sell alcohol there, but that didn't mean Bridgewater was a perfect little place. Like many small New England towns, Bridgewater could have been the setting for Grace Metalious's *Peyton Place*, and exposed similar small-town secrets. It was full of quaint colonial charm and judgmental gossip. Bridgewater had one general store, a post office, two banks, and no traffic lights. The annual volunteer firemen's country fair was held every August, complete with pig races, tractor pulls, lumberjack contests, and Jazzercise ladies wearing Spandex and plastered-on smiles.

My mom ran the Bridgewater Fair Art Show for 21 years. When I was nine, we all took over the running of the fair's Pet Parade. Even then, we were a little unusual. When we inherited the event, the categories included "Cutest Bunny" and "Most Beautiful Bird." My mom, Mic, and I put our own twist on things. Some of our new categories were "Pet with Best Breath" and "Pet with Longest Tongue." We supplied our judges with Craftsman measuring tapes, and they obediently took accurate measurements (though one year, we did have an uncooperative ferret).

We raised a Guiding Eyes for the Blind puppy named Gomer. We didn't give him this name. When a litter of potential guide-dog puppies is born, the names of all the puppies in the litter start with same first letter. Obviously, Gomer was in the "G" litter, and I think they were running out of names by the time he was born. All of us came to hate the phrase "Get busy," the mandatory code when you wanted the dog to pee or poop, but his graduation at Guiding Eyes headquarters made us all proud of the responsible dog we had raised.

We had a pot-bellied pig named Madeline, who we rescued from a family that bought her as a tiny pink piglet, but when she grew up, they kept her locked in a dog crate 24 hours a day. At our house, she slept on her favorite fluffy blanket in the kitchen every night, and wore a fluorescent green Invisible Fence collar that kept her on our property. We gave her baths in the bathtub, and would throw hunks of romaine lettuce into the water to distract her.

My parents decided to get chickens when I was four years old and Mic was in first grade. The main reason was because of the growing tick-borne Lyme disease problem, which had originated in Connecticut. Free-range chickens eat ticks, but they don't get Lyme disease, and it isn't passed on to their eggs, either. My dad converted our old outhouse (yes, we had an outhouse) into a chicken coop.

Dozens of chicks were incubated on the kitchen counter, as was a Greylag goose named Bronco, who imprinted onto Mic and followed him everywhere. Faye, our pygmy goat, butted everyone except Mic.

When Mic joined Poultry 4-H, my dad built a 14-nesting-box coop to his specifications. We gave every chicken old-fashioned names like Muriel, Gertrude, Bertha, Mildred, and Sarah. Mic and I took great pride in recording all kinds of useless information about them, and about future chickens, in a bound burgundy ledger with golden curlicues. I actually thought this treasured written record would be passed on to future generations in our family, and that every entry was as important and official as the town clerk's duties at town hall. Sadly, the ledger included chicken obituaries: *Betty (Rhode Island Red) died August 30, 1997—fox attack, Wilma (daughter of Doris) carried off by a hawk on November 26, 1997, Sally (Silver-Laced Wyandotte) disappeared on the night of October 11, 1998—we think the bobcat got her.*

We named our first rooster Stuart after our road, Stuart Road. Stuart wasn't one of those aggressive attack roosters. He'd let me carry him around, and hung out with me while I cooked meals on the plastic stove in the playhouse. When he found some tasty tidbit in the leaves, like a slug or a woolly bear, he'd call the hens over to share the bounty. All of us got to know what their cackles, crows, squawks, and cock-a-doodles meant: *I'm laying an egg. Wow, I just found a worm. Watch out, there's a squirrel in the tree. It's 4:20 A.M., hurry up and open the coop!*

One weekend, we took a two-night trip to Newport, Rhode Island, and left the chickens in the coop with plenty of food and water. When we got home on Sunday, I went up to the coop to check on the chickens and collect eggs. Sarah, alone at the end of the outdoor pen, seemed to be standing very still. When I got closer, I saw that her head was totally bitten off. Her neck, pulled through the chicken wire, was keeping her propped up.

My dad understood the story through my tears, and when we walked back to the coop together, he figured out that a raccoon or fox had bitten her head off as she was pecking outside the wire. Traumatized Stuart was crowing crazily and jumping in circles. I guess it would be similar to being locked in a room with your headless wife for 48 hours. When my dad opened the coop door, Stuart exploded out to the woods and didn't come home for five days. For the rest of his life, he was reluctant to go back in the coop at night.

When I tell people that I went to a K-5 elementary school with less than 100 students and only one of each grade, they think it sounds like a lovely one-room schoolhouse. It wasn't. Being with the same 20 kids for six years was monotonous. My class was particularly dysfunctional, and so much time was wasted on behavioral issues. In a larger school, the class dynamics are mixed up every year, and you're not stuck with the same people.

The thing that made my time at Burnham School bearable was my mom's weekly class. She became the elementary teacher for gifted students in our school district. People ask me if it was a weird experience to have my mom as a teacher, but honestly, it wasn't. I never went through that *everything my parents do is embarrassing* stage.

My mom was a very popular teacher because of her kooky personality, and her belief that learning should never be boring. Why look at prepared slides under a microscope when it's a lot more fun to examine your own (and even an agreeable principal's) earwax? The food chain and circle of life make more sense when you dissect an owl pellet and see bones from an owl's meal. Learning about ancient Egyptian mummification becomes much more exciting when you get to spend four weeks making your own mummy from a raw Perdue Oven-Stuffer Roaster (and somehow, there is no odor involved).

One year, my mom's second graders won first place in the National Statistical Association Poster Contest with the topic "Is your bellybutton concave or convex?" The kids made a pretty funny bar graph, and I'm sure they never forgot the definitions of the two words.

Whenever it was someone's birthday at my school, they would seek out my mom for one of her special forehead kisses. She would turn it into this elaborate event where she'd stop teaching to select just the right shade of Cover Girl Outlast lipstick from her purse (usually Wild Berry Wink) and apply a thick coat to her lips. She'd hold the kids' cheeks in her hands, dramatically kiss them on the forehead, and insist the kiss had to stay there all day. The kids would threaten to wipe them off, but they would proudly walk the halls, reminding me of colorful Ash Wednesday celebrants. Even the fifth graders would beg her for these badges of honor.

The last few minutes of each class, she would have everyone sit in a circle as she asked *Trivial Pursuit Junior* questions as a behavioral incentive. Each time a kid got a question right, they got a Skittle and a shrill "Ding! Ding! Ding!" from my mom. She had a talent for selecting questions tailored to each kid without being obvious, so that everyone would get a question right. But really, nobody cared about the Skittles. The thing they loved the most was the weekly candy story. I don't know how this ever started, but each week, my mom would come up with an outlandish disaster that had happened to the Skittles, which were always kept in a big plastic container in her green rolling teaching bag, which was always in the back of the Tahoe. Each week, she would weave the tale, and the more outrageous it was, the more her students believed it was true.

The stories ranged from the time Mic had left the car windows open in the car wash and the soapy foam got all over the candy, to when we went to the Capuchin Catacombs in Sicily and mummy powder got on the candy (do you really think she carted her teaching bag to Sicily?), to the time Mic accidentally ripped open a bag of chicken food and the pellets mixed with the Skittles in the open container.

Almost every made-up mishap was blamed on Mic, which added to the delight of her students. The kids were convinced that they could taste the soapy water, the mummy powder, or the chicken food. I know it sounds unbelievable that the kids fell for these stories, but my mom is a very convincing liar. I was the only student who knew the truth, and I never spilled the beans. She worked at the school for eight years, and never repeated a story.

None of my mom's students should feel bad that they were deceived, because she also lied to her own children. For years, Mic and I believed that she literally had eyes in the back of her head and could distinguish between different colors of M&Ms in her mouth without even looking at them. She couldn't. We eventually realized that she was sneaking a peek in the Victorian mirror that hung in our dining room as we placed an M&M on her tongue.

I now know that my mom thought mainstream disciplinary methods were not very effective. Because of this, she devised her own unique punishments. She told us that she had recorded a whole season of *Matlock* episodes on a VCR tape, and if we misbehaved, we would have to watch the whole thing. I didn't even know what *Matlock* was, but the name sounded kind of scary, like a show with creepy serial killers or kidnapped victims locked in basements. I never had any idea it was just a boring show about a folksy 1980s lawyer. Of course, it never occurred to Mic or me that she had no idea how to record a show. She could barely even turn on the VCR!

Velya

To me, things like "time-outs" and "the naughty corner" were pretty dopey. I mean, like, "the child should not be in time out for longer than one minute per year old that she is." That was way too much math for me, so I devised my own fool-proof punishment. The mere mention of it was guaranteed to end any squabble or bad behavior.

We had a vacuum cleaner called the *Fantom Fury,* which was a black-bagless-lightweight-upright vacuum cleaner. It came with on-board attachments that "easily fit into the hose/handle assembly." Its big selling feature was "you can see the dirt and dust swirling in the cyclonic canister as your carpets are cleaned," which I guess was supposed to be motivational. Along with the "long-lasting HEPA filter," the *Fantom Fury* also came with an informative videotape. I assume it was informative—I never watched it. Why would I want to? There are a lot of things in this world that get me excited:

a new batch of library books, Chanel No. 5, an income tax refund—but never a vacuum.

One day, when Ehris and Mic were arguing about whose turn it was to have to drink the gross clumpy stuff at the bottom of the Edensoy soy milk container (this is something they now insist I was always making them do, like an obsessed Gestapo agent who somehow also grew up during the Great Depression), I had a brainstorm. I calmly informed them that if they didn't knock it off, they would both have to watch the 30-minute *Fantom Fury* video, then take the accompanying quiz I had prepared in advance for just such an occasion. When your mother is a teacher, this quiz stuff is pretty believable. I implied that something really, really bad would happen if they did not pass the quiz.

It worked like a charm! They gulped down the soy milk, clumps and all, and kind of slithered out of the kitchen. I couldn't believe my brilliance!

I have to admit that both of our kids were generally extremely well-behaved. However, from time to time, they acted up and needed a reprimand—or, as I prefer to think of it, a little negative reinforcement.

Ehris

It's kind of unusual nowadays for kids to play outside, but when I was three years old, I spent hours in the woods outside our house, where my dad had hung a set of swinging rings in a tall maple tree. I would head out for the rings as if I were leaving for work, wearing my regular costume of high-top light-up sneakers and a bright purple leotard with an orange flounce around the legs, and pink bows and elaborate cutouts in the back. Everyone knew where I was going, and they let me do my thing.

My mom often packed me my favorite snack: a baggie of "fancy crackers" and a berry Juicy-Juice juice box ("fancy crackers" was what Mic and I called those hexagonal Oyster crackers that people put in soup).

At the tree, I would jump up, grab the black plastic rings, and swing and twirl. I pictured myself in a classy circus, kind of like Cirque du Soleil, as my curly tresses floated behind me and the orange flounce lifted and fluttered. My little palms were almost as calloused as my dad's, and I loved it.

At the time, around 1995, there was a very popular toy called a Sky Dancer. A little foam-winged plastic fairy was inserted into a pull-string base. When you pulled the string, she would launch into the air like a helicopter. My favorite Sky Dancer had blond hair in a high ponytail, and wore a purple sequined tutu and purple ballet shoes. Like Mic, who was convinced people really thought he was a zebra in his homemade Halloween costume (as in, "Wow, look at that zebra galloping around outside!"), I thought I looked exactly like my airborne purple sparkly Sky Dancer as I spun and swung. I felt free and without limits, which is the same way my family has always made me feel.

While my mom took care of the details in my family's life, we could all tell when my dad was cooking up something fun. He'd walk around with a measuring tape, check the *Bargain News*, make some phone calls, and not really pay attention to what was going on around him. Mic, my mom, and I would smile at each other with knowing glances when he would finally say, "You know, I was thinking...." We never had any idea what my dad was going to propose, but it was always something interesting.

My dad came up with the idea to buy a used white E-Z-Go gas-powered golf cart, which Mic and I drove for hours every day in the woods behind our house. We made golf-cart licenses out of Pop-Tart boxes, using our "picture day" photos from Burnham Elementary School. My dad would often come home from work and have to dislodge the golf cart from swamps, tree stumps, boulders, or mud, and didn't grumble about any of it. My parents thought that we could learn how to drive and crash into trees way before we would actually have our real licenses.

Mic and I rarely got into golf cart accidents, but there were a few exceptions. One afternoon, we had been driving the golf cart for a while, and decided to jazz things up a bit by creating a game called "Guess Where You Are!" I got into the driver's seat and closed my eyes. Mic sat in the passenger seat with his foot on the gas pedal, told me which way to turn, and had me guess where I was driving. Were we at Barn Hill, Bathroom Stop, Fox Mountain, the playhouse? I don't really know what happened, since I had my eyes closed, but I think Mic's size 15 sneaker somehow got caught on the gas pedal, accidentally pressing it to the floor.

Obviously, the golf cart was speeding through the woods. Following the rules of our game, I still had my eyes closed, and we hit a tree. I was launched forward, hit my ribs on the steering wheel, and was catapulted diagonally onto the ground. I was shaken up for a bit, but this didn't keep me from driving for long. Even today, Mic denies that the crash was his fault, so in full disclosure, one time I accidentally ran over his foot with the golf cart.

When my parents bought a used boat, all four of us took the mandatory boating course and received our boating licenses. At eight years old, I could legally drive anything up to a 45-foot yacht (as long as it wasn't for commercial use). We also got two used jet skis from the *Bargain News*, and my dad and Mic sank one of them in the middle of Candlewood Lake when they forgot to plug the drain hole.

My dad built us a treehouse high in the limbs of a hickory tree. Mic and I would load snacks like Goldfish, Zebra Cakes, or Cosmic Brownies into a metal bucket with a long rope tied to the handle. One of us would scamper up the treehouse ladder and hoist up the pail of goodies. One time, we were up in the treehouse and my dad was down on the ground, pretending to attack us. Our snack bucket was filled with hickory nuts, and we started brandishing it like a weapon. My dad had no idea that a swinging bucket of nuts was about to hit him in the forehead. I still remember the way he staggered and had to sit down on a log. I know now that Mic and I were more upset than he could ever be.

My parents make a pretty good pair. My dad has no idea when the dogs are due for rabies shots, he's never paid a cable bill, and since he always just picks the shirt on top, my mom has to regularly rearrange the shirts in his drawer. She could find the title to one of our cars in two seconds. He could tell you about its rocker arms, motor mounts, and pneumatic shocks. My mom knows his Social Security number, what Mic and I wore on the first day of kindergarten, and the last time the furnace was cleaned. My dad is always losing his yoga mat, and has nine pairs of cheapo magnifying reading glasses scattered all over the house because he never remembers where he leaves them.

One Saturday, he came home from doing a construction estimate. Sitting at the dining room table, he told us, "They seemed pretty interested, but they kept staring at me while I was talking."

My mom snorted, "Yeah, I'd stare at you, too! The plastic sticker that says what strength the glasses are is still stuck on the left lens!"

Sometimes I think of my mom, dad, and me as the circles in a Venn diagram. One circle contains my dad's steady peace, sense of adventure, and "all mistakes can be fixed" and "anything is possible" philosophies. My mom's circle is outgoing, nurturing, enthusiastic, and a lover of the arts. At the overlapping intersection are the traits all three of us share: open-mindedness, a sense of humor, and responsibility. From my remarkable parents, I've inherited all of those things.

CHAPTER EIGHT

Velya

After 15 years in the corporate world, Jim was traveling more and more for his job as a regional operations manager, and was about to move into the types of positions for which he could have been transferred anywhere in the United States. We were at a crossroads in our lives. At the time, we didn't like the prospect of moving, because we were content with our Bridgewater life. I encouraged Jim to take the leap and open his own construction business—or, as he would assert, *our* own business. We founded Urban Crossroads, Inc., a home remodeling company. Its success was largely due to its advertising slogan, "Simple Projects, Major Projects, *Impossible* Projects."

While other contractors were interested in building only McMansions, cathedral-ceiling great rooms, or high-end kitchens for couples with disposable incomes, Jim was willing to tackle any project, from installing a dryer vent, hanging wallpaper, or refurbishing a pool house to designing and constructing an authentic-looking addition for a colonial home.

Few people have the dedication it takes to be self-employed. Jim, however, excelled at being his own boss, because he expected more from himself than anyone else ever could have. It's been said that someone's weakest quality is their strongest quality carried to an extreme. Jim held himself to the highest of standards.

Jim could figure out how to renovate just about anything, and wasn't afraid to make a mistake or ask for help. We bought and successfully flipped several houses. One of them was in such a state of disrepair that even Habit for Humanity wasn't interested in it. It had become a crack house, and squatters had burned the wooden stairs leading to the basement for heat. Jim had no qualms about asking questions at the plumbing store, hardware store, quarry, tile store, or hardwood flooring place. He willingly accepted suggestions and advice from old guys, furnace guys, heat duct guys, well guys, septic guys, plumbing guys, all kinds of guys.

To understand Jim, you have to know him. He's the kind of guy you'd want with you during a hijacking, on the Titanic, or at the natural birth of your nine-pound eight-ounce firstborn (as he was), but he's also the kind of guy who never missed an open house, parent-teacher conference, spring concert, night of trick-or-treating, or voice recital. He makes you feel like nothing is too hard to accomplish, and all mistakes can be fixed.

Every morning, he sits on the edge of our bed and stares out the bedroom window, thinking, thinking, thinking. "Five minutes, Jim. Just five minutes. That's how long I'd love to be in your brain and see what actually goes on in there," I used to say fairly frequently. I envisioned a peppy hamster jogging on one of those metal exercise wheels, sometimes running so fast that wood chips scattered everywhere. In the case of a real hamster, of course, running as fast as it could would get it nowhere. In Jim's case, he was always formulating a project—never a scheme, but an idea.

It wasn't until 28 years into our marriage that I stopped asking Jim what he was thinking about as he sat on the bed and concentrated. It wasn't that I didn't care—it just took me that long to realize he wouldn't vocalize the idea until he was ready. Jim always ran his ideas past me before acting upon them. All the days and all the years of the two of us together, we have been a team.

CHAPTER NINE

Ehris

The seeds of change can be planted unexpectedly. I was four years old, and my dad was building a stone wall down by the lake at my grandparents' house. That was when we met Jose Geraldo Martins Bastos Teixeira from Abre Campo, Brazil. My dad needed help building the wall, but his usual workers were busy. Someone suggested Jose, who had just arrived in the United States and was looking for work.

My mom, Mic, and I were there that day, and we ordered pizza for lunch. My dad stopped working and invited Jose to come up to the patio and eat with us. Jose spoke only a few words of English, and said quietly, "No, thank you, I finish build wall."

"Jose, come eat with us!" my mom coaxed.

After declining a few more times, he eventually conceded, "Okay, I eat lunch." Although we didn't speak Portuguese and he didn't speak English, we all tried so hard to understand each other. My dad and Jose hit it off, and began to work together more and more frequently. Every night at dinner, my dad would entertain us with Jose's latest stories, which all began, "Jeem, you no believe!" It would take days for my dad to hear these entire tales, because Jose would begin telling the story, start laughing, and then be unable to finish.

My favorite story (which Jose always told the exact same way, sprinkled with hearty laughter) was about Margaret. "One day," he said, "I meet a monkey. She very nice. She with organ grinder guy. He say to me, 'Jose, never give banana to Margaret.' But I like this monkey *so* much. I see her every day. I love her. I take banana from my home, hide it from my mother, run to Margaret. She grab banana from me, I happy, then she bite my arm. I shake my arm, she no let go, her tooths in my arm, I scream, she scream, organ grinder guy throw monkey snack on ground and she let go. It hurt *so* much!" Jose would roll up his sleeve and urge, "Come, look, see my scar!" A few months after hearing the story, my mom came across a pair of white socks with monkeys and bananas all over them at TJ Maxx. She gave them to Jose, and years later found out that he kept them in a special drawer.

Once, when my dad and Jose were replacing clapboard siding on an 18th-century house, Jose said to him, "Jeem, you no believe this story," and proceeded to tell him another one of his tales. Jose's uncle João had a big farm (over 250 hectares) with many rivers, ponds, and lakes. One summer, when Jose was a teenager, Uncle João called him and said he had a problem. "What's the problem?" Jose questioned. Uncle João was frantic. There was an alligator in the lake! Fearing for the safety of his calves, Uncle João asked Jose to come over and help him get the alligator out of the lake.

As a teenage boy, Jose was thrilled at the opportunity for some excitement. He galloped his mule over to Uncle João's farm, and they headed over to the lake where the alligator was lurking. Uncle João disappeared and came back holding a 12-gauge shotgun. He pointed to the rowboat on the shore and said to Jose, "*Boa sorte!*" (Good luck!). Jose thought, *Man, what have I gotten myself into?* Wanting to keep up his *machismo* (a Latin American thing that identifies men with authority and strength, and women with weakness and subservience), he grabbed the gun, pushed the boat off the shore, and hopped in. Jose rowed out into the middle of the lake and waited. Suddenly, a big pair of nostrils emerged from the murky water. Jose was both terrified and excited. He pulled the trigger and was thrown backward from the force. The bullet grazed the alligator's snout. Enraged, it leaped from the murky water into the boat! As the alligator jumped into the boat, Jose jumped into the lake. Since Jose could never make it through any story without cracking up uncontrollably, we never found out what happened to the alligator in Uncle João's lake.

Jose and my dad developed a very strong brotherly relationship. Before he met my dad, Jose had barely been making minimum wage. Many American contractors take advantage of immigrants, but my dad made sure Jose was paid every week. After working together for many months, my dad offered to show him how to do estimates, where to buy materials, how to talk to customers, and what to charge them. Jose was able to open his own construction company within a year, and supplied my dad with the workers he needed. My dad gave Jose many referrals, and offered him lucrative jobs when he was busy and couldn't get to them.

Velya

Jose would often send money back to Brazil, buy a small farm, sell it for a profit, and then buy another larger farm. He never saw these farms; they were just a means to an end.

Once, Jim raced home and proposed, "I think we should help Jose. He needs $15,000, or he's going to lose the farm in *Dores de Campos*. He said he'll work for me for free until he pays off the loan. Whaddaya think?"

We had periodically loaned Jose money if a farm payment was due, and he always paid back the debt. "That's a lot of money, Jim, but I know how important it is to him and Isabela," I said, writing out the check. Our families had become very close, and friends help friends. True to his word, Jose repaid the debt.

Jim and Jose worked together on a daily basis for eight years. Eventually, Jose and Isabela found the gigantic farm they had been looking for in a town called Ponte Nova. They planned for over a year, and finally moved back to Brazil. As happy as we were for Jose, we missed him terribly.

Soon after they settled in, Jose called and said, "Jeem, you all come see my house. We go horse riding, milk my cows, eat *churrasco* (barbequed meat). I show you my country." We jumped at his invitation to visit.

Years before, we had begun traveling on every school vacation and major holiday. When Jim and I got married on Thanksgiving weekend and then left for our honeymoon, we set a precedent of not being around for his parents' tense and uncomfortable family gatherings. My family was small: just my mother, father, Jordan, and me. By the time Jordan was a teenager, he had become a professional musician, and always had holiday gigs. So, although we celebrated with my parents and brother, it was never on the official date.

Jim and I hoped that by traveling and experiencing more than white-bread Bridgewater, the kids would be open to other cultures and ideas, free from prejudice and narrow-mindedness. We weren't by any means wealthy, but we had seen most of the United States by the time Ehris reached third grade, and began to travel internationally. As soon as we got home from one trip, we all looked forward to planning the next. In a good way, home felt very far away when I heard the call to prayer from a mosque's minaret in Morocco, or as we stood in front of the white marble tombs of Tsar Nicholas, his wife Alexandra, and their children in St. Petersburg.

Many people asked me if I felt guilty about not giving our children traditional holiday memories. People automatically assume that we're Christian, and have actually been aghast when they find out we don't put up a Christmas tree, Christmas lights, or Christmas stockings. There should be a term for people who don't believe in God as a guy sitting up in the clouds who created the world in seven days, but *do* believe that everything is comprised of energy that cannot be created or destroyed. My mother always worshipped the wonder of Mother Nature.

When I was growing up, Christmas, which included gift-giving, was simply a celebration of winter. Easter, complete with baskets and Easter egg hunts, was a celebration of spring. My mother raised us under her umbrella of beliefs—a mix that included being a good person simply because it's the right thing, a respect for the Earth and other people's

54

beliefs, and the preciousness of life. We ate wheat germ and yogurt, and didn't smash spiders. We rescued earthworms who surfaced after rainstorms and helped snapping turtles cross the road. Our Ford Torino station wagon, driven by my wacky mom, often became the getaway car for mice captured in our basement. We unlatched the Havahart traps in nearby fields as the astonished mice scampered to freedom.

Way back during Jim's days at Saint Rose of Lima School in Newtown, he had already begun to dislike the hypocrisy of Catholicism. So, we passed on to our kids the same concepts my mom had passed on to Jordan and me. If I had to label myself, I guess I'm an open-minded atheist with a moral compass that points north, and I believe that no one but me directs my fate.

Once, before a faculty meeting, someone asked what we had done for Thanksgiving. When I said that we had eaten turkey club sandwiches at a Denny's in Maine, some of the women at the conference room table looked at me with a combination of pity and disgust. People have actually chided, "How can you do that to your children? What kind of mother are you?" Back then, I worried too much about making other people feel bad, so I never would have said what I *really* wanted to say: *Why is it okay for you to criticize the way I celebrate the holidays, but I don't make any judgment about the way you do? Does it really matter how, or where, or if, you celebrate?*

Jim and I never lied to the kids about the existence of Santa Claus, the Easter Bunny, or the Tooth Fairy. We believed this insulted the intelligence of children, and were honest with Mic and Ehris. When they asked, we answered, "Do you think there could *really* be a man who flies around in a sleigh and delivers presents to every single kid in the world on one night?" Jim and I simply said that these were games mommies and daddies played with their kids. They seemed satisfied with this explanation, and never ruined the fiction for other kids.

As Mic and Ehris lost their baby teeth, they put them under their pillows. They would wake to find a letter from Toothie, which usually included a scavenger hunt for their reward. I couldn't bear the thought of just throwing their baby teeth away, so I saved them in two pink and gold vintage Avon perfume jars. Actually, I also have my own baby teeth in a white and lime green Avon jar.

It's not that we're anti-holiday. As a matter-of-fact, our kids always made handmade gifts for family, friends, and teachers. There were the clove-studded tangerine pomanders tied up in plastic netting onion bags, which we collected for seven months. They made golden spray-painted elbow macaroni jewelry boxes, and caterpillar clothespin pom-pom magnets. All of their Halloween costumes were homemade, including Mic's kangaroo costume. Mic took great pride in telling people that his tail was stuffed with "Daddy's old underwear." One year, Mic and Ehris dressed up as Steve and Terri Irwin (you know, the Crocodile Hunter), and Ehris was once an adorable Nancy Drew.

I think we'd all say that we have created some pretty fabulous holiday memories on our own. Riding the funicular in Capri, strolling through the Frankfurt Christmas markets, taking a horse-drawn sleigh ride in Salzburg (with the driver in an authentic wolf suit), and the overnight ferry from Sweden to Finland were just some of the experiences we will never forget. We have also enjoyed a variety of

New Year's Eve celebrations: eating 12 grapes at the stroke of midnight on the Plaza Mayor in Spain, breathtaking fireworks in Taormina, Italy, while being doused in champagne, and the unforgettable night in Budapest when everyone, including the police, shot bottle rockets and fireworks in the street. Mic's face when he realized he had shot out a streetlight, and Ehris's reaction when a guy in a monkey suit jumped out in front of her on the sidewalk, make *Dick Clark's New Year's Rockin' Eve* and the dropping of the ball in Times Square seem pretty tame.

CHAPTER TEN

Ehris

That December, we were granted our five-year tourist visas, and took a two-week trip to Brazil. As a 12-year-old, I loved seeing the contrasts between North and South America. In Rio de Janeiro and São Paulo, we saw all the predictable tourist attractions, like Sugarloaf Mountain, Christ the Redeemer, Ipanema, and Copacabana. I was amazed by the power of Iguassu Falls, bordering Brazil, Argentina, and Paraguay. On a seventh-grade field trip to Hyde Park, our tour guide said that when Eleanor Roosevelt laid eyes on Iguassu Falls, she exclaimed, "Poor Niagara!" Niagara Falls is amazing, but Iguassu Falls is untamed. There aren't any fences or gates to keep you from getting close to Iguassu, and it's a lot less commercialized. There are acres of protected forest and nature trails. At our hotel, we ate breakfast on the terrace overlooking the falls while *koatimundi* sneakily snatched papaya and *pão de queijo* from us.

Many people don't realize that Brazil is about the size of the United States. We took a flight to our next stop: Jose and Isabela's 300-acre dairy farm in Ponte Nova.

We hadn't seen Jose for about a year and a half. He picked us up at the airport in Belo Horizonte on Christmas Day, and my mom didn't stop asking questions during the whole three-hour ride to their house—but that was nothing new. She asked stuff like, "Do you have electricity? Do you have running water? Do you have a microwave?"

Jose laughed to himself and responded simply, "You'll see." Hundreds of coconut palms lined the dirt road that led to Jose's farm. It was like a scene from *National Geographic*. Cows and horses grazed in the fields, green parrots with yellow faces hopped around in the branches of mango trees, and football-sized papayas lay where they had dropped along the driveway. Secluded in the green mountains was the apricot-colored stucco house with a clay tile roof. Isabela and their 11 year-old son, Matheus, were waiting for us by the pool.

Entering the house, we were greeted by two maids wearing white caps who had prepared a traditional American Christmas feast. It was weird to be in a Brazilian-style house and be surrounded by American appliances. Brazil and the United States have the same electric current, so all the appliances from Jose and Isabela's house in Connecticut worked in the new house. Max, the Springer Spaniel they had gotten as a puppy in Connecticut, rolled over and waited for his usual belly rub from me.

Like most Americans, we didn't know anything about Brazil. We imagined there would be anacondas and jaguars lurking around. Jose and Isabela had two tiny white poodles.

"You leave them out all night?" my mom gasped. "Nothing eats them?"

"Yes, I no lie to you." Jose chuckled.

"Oh, man! Imagine if we left Chauncey outside all night in Connecticut?" She laughed. "He'd be gobbled up by a fox, bobcat, or coyote in a heartbeat!"

Even though there were deadly snakes and other creepy animals in Brazil, Jose told us, "The first time I ever see anaconda was New York City, in the Bronx Zoo."

CHAPTER ELEVEN

Ehris

O n our second day with Jose and Isabela, they asked us
if we'd like to see the city of Ouro Preto (Black Gold),
a UNESCO site and the focus of Brazil's gold rush from the
1690s to the late 1800s. In Ouro Preto, slaves had worked
the mines and lived under cruel conditions. As soon as we
arrived, guides rushed over to the car and offered to give us
tours. My dad and Jose made arrangements with a guy who
led us down winding cobblestone streets, past brightly colored houses, and into the old mine. We all posed for a photo
in front of the mine entrance, wearing white paper shower
caps under bright orange construction helmets. I can't look
at that photo anymore.

As they had been at Iguassu Falls, safety precautions at
this abandoned gold mine were pretty nonexistent. We were
given orange plastic helmets, but the muddy rock tunnel
wasn't braced up with any kind of support. All of us (except
for my five-foot-tall mom) kept smashing our heads on the
stone ceiling. We learned that they castrated all the slaves
except for one short man, who had fathered all the slave
babies. This way, all of the children would be short enough

to work in the mine without slowing down work quotas by having to duck. The slaves couldn't escape; they had been permanently chained together. At the end of the cave, there was a pile of picks and shovels. We each grabbed a tool and got a very brief taste of life in the mine—minus the chains, brutality, and castration. During the mine tour, we learned that slaves smuggled gold out of the mines under their fingernails and in tooth cavities. They made offerings to the church by rinsing their hair in the holy water, leaving behind little flakes of gold.

On the dusty dirt road back to Ponte Nova, Jose slammed on the brakes. As my forehead smashed into the front headrest, Isabela shouted, "Jeem, Jeem, get the *maracujá*! It's on the floor!" My dad was clueless about what was happening, and what a *maracujá* could be.

The day before, Jose had hit the brakes, yelling, "Jeem, Jeem, get out of the truck and get the *tatu*!" My dad leapt out of the front seat and started running down the dirt road in his Docksiders and khaki shorts, not sure what he was after. He glanced over his shoulder and saw Jose trotting down the road after him, pointing at something. Jose called, "Quick, Jeem! It's getting away!"

My dad saw what Jose was pointing at, and realized he was chasing an armadillo. As he caught the baby armadillo, it peed on his hand in terror. After we all had a chance to pet it, Jose gently placed the *tatu* in the weeds on the side of the road.

By now, my dad was pretty used to this hopping-out-of-the-truck routine. This time, he was after a *maracujá* (passion fruit) that had fallen out of a tree and landed on the *chão*, which is the Portuguese word for both *ground* and *floor*. We never really knew what was happening when we went on these outings with Jose.

Comparing Connecticut to Brazil is like comparing New England apple crisp to South American *pudim de mango*. They're both delicious, but very different. At Brazilian tollbooths, the attendants gave out candy. Mayonnaise came in a variety of flavors, and though the brand was Hellman's, the options were regular, light, lime, lemon, tuna, tomato, salsa, red onion, ham, garlic, *churrasco*, chive, olive oil, and cheese. Motels were just for sex. Hardly anyone had hot water at their kitchen or bathroom sinks, and the only hot water in the house was in the shower. Most people had a soaker machine to soak dirty laundry *before* it went in the washing machine, since the red clay dirt was very hard to wash out of clothes. A paper towel and napkin brand was called "Snob." Everyone wore white or silver on New Year's Eve. Pizza came in a 12-sided box and was topped with corn, olives, ham, and hard-boiled eggs, with a crust the consistency of hamburger buns. *Arroz e feijão* (rice and beans) were served at every lunch and dinner, every day. The cashiers at grocery stores sat down, and instead of plastic order dividers, they often used sticks. Potatoes came in two varieties: clean and dirty. All of this just added to what we were starting to love about Brazil.

One day, we stopped at what I thought was a tire shop. Jose turned off the ignition and said, "Jeem, come try. We all eat lunch here."

We followed Jose and Isabela through a stacked-tire fortress, which opened onto a pond surrounded by two gigantic outdoor fish tanks, an ancient swing set, and a building that seemed to be falling down. A thin gray-haired man in jeans, work boots, and a fluorescent orange shirt popped out of the tire fortress to greet us. He introduced himself as the owner of this *Pesque e Pague*, and told Jose he was delighted to meet Americans.

Isabela, who spoke much better English than Jose, explained, "*Pesque e Pague* means Fish and Pay. It's very popular in Brazil, especially in Minas Gerais. People bring fishing poles and go fishing in the pond. If you catch a fish, you can throw it back or pay to take it home. You can only throw the fish back in the pond if it's not hurt. You can bring it home whole, or he can take out the guts."

The owner caught a big tilapia for us. He brought it inside the building, and his daughter helped clean and prepare it for frying. We all huddled around a rusty metal table under an umbrella to get out of a sudden downpour. The *Pesque e Pague* owner appeared, proudly carrying two plates of fish with lime wedges. His daughter kept us well supplied with fresh *suco de cajú* (cashew fruit juice) as the rain made a moat around the table. The weather could have made this a miserable meal, but being with good friends in a new situation made this a lunch I'll never forget.

The next morning at the farm, we got up at dawn. Jose gave each of us a pair of rubber boots and handed me a straw hat and a lasso. "Now you a cowgirl!" he laughed. We all followed Jose to the milking parlor. Two farm hands were in the pasture rounding up the cows, who were willingly making their way down to the corral, since their udders were full and they wanted relief. Each cow waited patiently in line until her turn came. Many dairy farmers in Brazil still liked to milk by hand, even though there were milking machines available. Jose's workers milked by hand in one corral, and by machine in the other. Brazilian cows kind of look like black and white Holsteins, but with a hump like a Brahma bull. Somehow, this hump helps them tolerate the intense heat. Their ears flop down like a goat's, unlike those of a typical cow in the United States.

Jose patted a massive black and white cow on the rump and said, "This cow, she name *Formiga*. She good cow. She give 15 to 20 liters milk every day. In Brazil, for taking milk, we let the baby drink from the *mamãe* just to make milk come out. Then, we take the milk until she almost dry. Then the baby suck the rest."

Brazilian farmers don't use a milking stool. Instead, they sit on something they construct with two small two-by-fours nailed into a T shape. They manage to balance on it while milking a 1,200-pound animal. Almost all Brazilian farmers, including Jose, either wear flip-flops (*Havaianas,* of course) or bare feet while in the corral. This is dangerous, because their feet could be stomped upon; also, the mud and cow poop are so deep that it's over the ankles of the workers, oozing between their toes. *Bicho de pé*, a parasitic insect that burrows into the soles of the feet or under the toenails, is very common. *Bicho de pé* literally means "bug of foot."

The workers would arrive at the corral in white rubber boots (at every farm we visited, the boots were always white), but they always took them off while working. I don't think it had anything to do with money, because Jose could have afforded any kind of boots. It was just one of the many Brazilian things we could never get properly explained, just like the way they couldn't understand why Americans allow pets in the house. The symptoms of *bicho de pé* include itchy feet and dirty toenails, so I was a little paranoid at every itch.

Formiga was led into the milking parlor. Rodrigo, the worker, tied her tail and back legs together with an old rope, so he wouldn't be kicked or swished in the face by her tail. He motioned for my dad to come and try his hand at milking. None of us had milked a cow before, so this was a dream come true for my dad. He put his calloused hands on Formiga's teats and started squeezing. Nothing happened. Rodrigo bent over to give him a short lesson in Portuguese. He eventually got a few dribbles of milk, but when Jose took over, the steaming milk gushed out like water from a hose. My mom, Mic, and I each tried, and the results weren't any better than my dad's. I'll never look at the gallons of milk at Stop & Shop in the same way!

CHAPTER TWELVE

Velya

Ever since we had begun traveling, all four of us dreamed of one day living in a foreign country. Once in Brazil, we fell in love with the country, culture, and people. We delighted in all of it, and the images still come to me like photographs behind my eyelids. The little pots of rubber cement at the post office to brush glue on envelopes and stamps. The huge clumps of weeds placed in the road instead of orange traffic cones to indicate an accident. Enormous ice cream cones in flavors like papaya, passion fruit, corn, and coconut pineapple. Riding bareback down dirt roads as the breeze rattled the sugarcane. Cows with muzzles that turned a foamy orange from the juicy mangoes they picked from the ground. I marveled at the way the cows spit out the hairy pits. The chunks of milk bobbing like buoys at the top of a cup of strong coffee. The hospitality.

While Jim and Jose repaired some fences at the farm, Ehris, Mic, and I decided to venture out into the center of Ponte Nova, about 20 minutes away from Jose and Isabela's house. I think Isabela was pretty sure she'd never see us again. I'm surprised she didn't pin their address and phone number onto our T-shirts, like kindergarteners on the first day of school. We took the bus to a *papelaria* (paper store), where we bought postcards. There, Ehris asked if anyone knew of a good hair salon. All of these actions sound pretty simple, but very few people speak English in rural Brazil. An old lady, whose name we later found out was Betchy, proceeded to lead us across the street and into a tiny, dark parking garage. Mic, who was 14, whispered, "You know what it smells like in here? Sharpies and a fart!" He was right.

In retrospect, it was pretty stupid to have followed this old lady, but she looked harmless. Betchy led us up a flight of curved worn marble stairs, and I was shocked when we emerged into a beauty salon. Using her handy Portuguese/English dictionary (which wasn't so handy after all, because it lacked the word for "layers"), 12-year-old Ehris asked for a haircut and was taken into the adjoining room.

We expected that Betchy would leave after escorting us into the second-story beauty parlor. However, she stayed and hung out with Mic and me for over an hour. In addition to giving us her cell phone number, she showed us pictures of her very pregnant granddaughter, and unwound her graying bun. It went below her *bunda* (butt), and she told us she had friends with hair down to their feet. They were not allowed to cut their hair for some religious reason.

Obviously, there was a lot of gesturing and *wow*ing involved in this story, and I was getting mental images of Brazilian Cousin Its! She hovered over us like a protective mother hen and told everyone in the salon, everyone who entered the salon, and everyone in the waiting area that we were Americans she had found in the street. At least, I think this is what she said, since I didn't know any Portuguese. Mic, who thought he could understand Portuguese because he spoke Spanish, insisted that Betchy had said something about being a female knight and a seamstress who crafted shirts out of hair. Both Mic and I did a lot of nodding and smiling. I was beginning to wonder where they had taken Ehris, and actually asked Mic if he thought there was a back exit to the place. He didn't seem too concerned.

Walter, the owner of the salon, invited Mic and me deeper into the beauty parlor so that he could "get to know us better." This was nowhere near as creepy as it sounds. At this point, Betchy left. Walter told Mic stories about President Lula and the Pope (more nodding and smiling) as the women getting haircuts and dye jobs smiled and stared. It wasn't until that moment that I realized I was probably one of about four women in Brazil with short hair, and my hair was short and choppy even by American standards. I had no idea what these ladies were thinking, but I bet the word spread quickly that Americans were in town.

Ehris finally appeared. Her curly hair had been slightly trimmed and straightened with a blow dryer. It sort of resembled the 1960s signature hairstyle known as the flip, and she looked like a cross between Mary Tyler Moore, Condoleeza Rice, and a Miss America beauty pageant contestant. Ehris's loose curls were gone, replaced by hair that did not move. Her shoulder-length hair was backcombed slightly at the top, and now curled saucily out at the ends. She looked very Brazilian, and everyone in the salon gushed over her.

During the haircut, I counted the bills in my shorts pocket and said to Mic, "Oh man. I hope I have enough money with me!" Ehris's haircut turned out to be ten *real*, the equivalent of four dollars in the United States. On the bus back to Jose and Isabela's house, Ehris thought it was pretty funny that the wind coming through the windows didn't blow her hair around at all.

Ehris

On trail rides in the United States, the horses are usually chubby mares who know the route and can't wait to get back to the barn for dinner. There's no skill necessary on the part of the rider. In Brazil, riding horses is very laid back. When we went horseback riding at Jose and Isabela's house, I was wearing bright yellow Havaiana flip-flops, my mom had on denim shorts and Isabela's leather riding boots, my dad wore jeans, and Mic had on a blue bathing suit and bare feet. None of us wore helmets. Brazilians would laugh at helmets. The horse they brought out for my dad wasn't actually a horse. She was a grayish mule named *Cueca*, which means "Underwear." Isabela explained that this mule was the color of Jose's underwear in the United States. *Why is Jose's underwear a different color in the United States than in Brazil?* I wondered. Mic was on a little reddish pony named *Canela* (Cinnamon), and I chose Jacques, an old palomino horse. My mom was on a tick-infested painted pony called Rolph, whom they had borrowed from a neighbor. I'm not kidding about him being tick-infested. Connecticut (the home of Lyme disease) is famous for its ticks, but these bloated brown Brazilian ticks were very creepy as they waved and wiggled their exceptionally long legs.

Mic had a little trouble controlling Cinnamon, and my dad yelled, "Mic, you have to control your horse!" (ironic foreshadowing). Cinnamon, Mic, Jacques, and I went ahead of the group. Jose, on Iceberg, and my dad, on Underwear, followed. My mom's sedate horse, Rolph, made frequent stops for sugarcane and mangoes, and Isabela lagged behind to keep her company, occasionally slapping Rolph with a sugar cane switch to make him move. He was unfazed.

It's pretty funny to watch a horse eat a mango. They put the entire thing in their mouth, somehow peel it with their teeth, suck out the fruit, which covers their rubbery lips with foamy orange juice, and spit out the peel and the pit.

Underwear had had many homes before she came to live with Jose. My dad, who had never ridden a *mula* before, looked petrified when it came to crossing the narrow, rickety, holey wooden bridge marking the end of Jose's property. Jose gave him advice: "Jeem! Don't let Underwear go in the middle of bridge or it break and you fall in the *heever!*" (river). My dad just kind of held on and hoped for the best. As Underwear rounded the corner after the bridge, her hairy ears perked up as she recognized one of her former homes. She started to turn her head to the right, but Jose warned, "No, Jeem! Pull her head to left! Don't let her go! She's heading for the *heever!*" My dad tried with all of his strength, but Underwear knew who was in control. She jerked her head to the right and took off down a narrow dirt alley. People watching started to scream, laugh, or run. My dad was struggling, unsuccessfully, to control Underwear.

Underwear located her former house and stuck her big gray mule head right through the window (windows in Brazilian country homes don't have glass or screens; there's just a hole). The residents were at the kitchen table eating lunch, and when they saw the giant head, they shrieked in terror and ran for cover. My dad tried to tell them in English to stay calm and not scream, but of course they had no idea what this crazy American guy was saying. When it was all over, the whole village—babies, grandparents, dogs, kids with pacifiers, chickens, and toothless farmers—lined the dirt road, giggling and recounting what had happened.

Once my mom and pokey, tick-covered Rolph caught up to everybody, Mic said that he had been having a hard time controlling Cinnamon, as all she wanted to do was gallop. My dad couldn't understand why Mic, who'd had six years of horseback-riding lessons, was having so much difficulty with this little red pony. He finally grumbled, "Mic, if you can't control your horse, I'll trade with you. I'll take Cinnamon, you go on Underwear." Mic was thankful to be done with Cinnamon, and he snickered as they switched horses.

Whenever we go horseback riding in the United States, they bring out friendly, normal-size horses for Mic, my mom, and me. Then there's always a delay as they prepare my dad's horse. What they bring out of the barn is always a Clydesdale or Percheron named Hercules, Zeus, or Apollo. My dad isn't fat, but he is a big guy. I was concerned when he got on poor little Cinnamon that she would collapse with him on her back. Jose and Isabela reassured me that although Cinnamon was small, she was strong (they told us later that she was also pregnant!). My dad, Mic, and I mounted our horses and started down the dirt road. My mom was still on dawdling Rolph, and Isabela plodded along with her. Jose had already taken off on Iceberg, galloping through the Brazilian jungle on a shortcut to their farm. For some reason, he needed to get the keys to their car and drive it to a neighbor's house.

A few minutes into the ride, Cinnamon started acting up. She wanted to trot, but my dad instructed sternly, "No,

Cinnamon! We are just going to walk." Cinnamon shook her head wildly in rebellion. She started lifting each hoof high off the ground, and pawed the red dirt road like an irate bull. Meanwhile, Mic was on Underwear, who had just spotted another one of her former homes, and took off down a vine-canopied dirt road.

Cinnamon pulled against the reins and tried with all of her pony might to free her head from my dad's strong clutches. He was thinking, *If I can just manage to keep her head up so high that she can't see the ground, she'll calm down and won't be able to run.* He underestimated that little red pony. Even though he was pulling her head up so high that she couldn't possibly see where she was going, she still pawed the ground like a caged animal and started to gallop as fast as she could. It was pretty funny to watch my dad's struggle with Cinnamon as she took off down the road surrounded by rustling sugarcane, head held high, chestnut mane flowing.

After a few minutes of galloping, Cinnamon hadn't slowed her pace at all (actually, my dad claims she sped up). He realized in horror that his saddle was slipping sideways because it hadn't been cinched tightly enough. He was terror-stricken that he was going to wind up under Cinnamon with his feet stuck in the stirrups. My dad (who never stops thinking) calculated that if she slowed down enough so that he could get his legs over the saddle and jump off, he would be okay. Unfortunately, this was not going to happen. Stubborn Cinnamon was still galloping at full speed, foaming at the mouth. My dad swears that he was momentarily blinded by some of the foam. His olive green Brazilian canvas cowboy hat flew off and landed in a muddy puddle, but that was the least of his problems.

Jose suddenly appeared driving the car, and realized my dad was in trouble. He stopped the silver Fiat in the middle of the road, blocking Cinnamon's path. She had no choice but to slow down. My dad pulled her head even higher, and she finally stopped, panting heavily, eyeballs popping out, sweaty foam all over her chest. He quickly swung his legs over and jumped down before she could leap over the car and take off again. Jose gave my dad the keys to the car as he hopped on Cinnamon. She meekly behaved herself, and my dad could almost hear the pony's mocking laugh.

I rode up on dusty Jacques and grinned mischievously. "Do you want your hat back?"

Mic reappeared from his adventure with Underwear, heard what had happened, and smirked. "Oh, so you had a little trouble controlling Cinnamon?" After recovering from the incident, my dad laughed and retold the story with broad hand gestures and flailing arms—countless times, to anyone who would listen. It didn't matter if they didn't understand English.

CHAPTER THIRTEEN

Velya

❋

"Jeem, I say to you, you no believe this place," Jose said, telling us about a nearby *hotel fazenda*, Brazil's version of a dude ranch. "Nobody live there. We go on horse. Maybe *you* live there."

I had never considered moving to Brazil, but once we rode up to the *hotel fazenda* and saw what a place it must have been in its day, a possibility ignited.

To say it needed work was an understatement. It was a run-down Brazilian colonial estate with a huge *varanda*, an antique wrought-iron gate, lots of rooms, a jungle treehouse, and loads of potential charm. It was the kind of place Jim could have transformed into a paradise. I saw myself floating around the *varanda*, offering guests chilled *caipirinhas* and looking glamorously tropical in a flowy sundress—not the sweaty mess I always seemed to be in August in Connecticut.

The hardest I have ever laughed was on our last night in Brazil. Somehow, we all wound up on the tile floor of Jose and Isabela's laundry room. Having been on many tour-type vacations, I knew tourists would fall in love with the charming *hotel fazenda*. Tourists eat up local color and traditional ways of life, but they also want their hot showers, Wi-Fi, and scrambled eggs with buttered white toast.

Jose and Isabela couldn't see the attraction of rural Brazilian life. Isabela narrowed her eyes and asked, "Why would someone want to bounce around in a dirty mule cart on a muddy road?"

"You guys don't get it," I explained. "That's exactly how New Englanders feel about stuff like apple orchards, stone walls, and fall foliage. It's everyday life to us, so we don't notice or appreciate it. To people who don't live in Brazil, things like bird of paradise growing wild, loaded mango trees, and turquoise parrots are exotic and exciting."

As Jim, Ehris, Mic, and I became more and more excited about the idea, Jose and Isabela caught our contagious enthusiasm. We all imagined how much fun it could be to own the *hotel fazenda* as a tourist vacation destination.

"We could take the guests on trail rides and river rafting," Mic said.

"And how about slow rides in mule carts for the less adventurous guests?" I suggested.

Ehris offered, "We could go monkey and *koatimundi* spotting!"

Jim added, "And take day trips to the old gold mine in *Ouro Preto*."

"Oh my god, you guys, I have the best idea! You know how those tours always offer optional excursions?" I asked. Turning to Jose and Isabela, I continued, "We could offer an optional evening excursion to your farm and advertise it like this: At *Fazenda Granja do Bamba*, you will have the opportunity to step back in time and interact with real-live Brazilians. Familiarize yourself with life, the way it used to be."

Ehris giggled, "That's exactly how those descriptions sound!"

"Oh my god!" I shrieked, rolling around on the laundry room floor. "I'm cracking myself up! Hey Jose, here's what you have to do! In bare feet and wearing some indigenous costume, whatever *that* is, you could rush out to the *varanda* and greet your guests with a heartily accented, 'Good evening. Come in, come in!'"

Isabela smiled, "Fatima and I could be hard at work at the *fogão a lenha*...."

"Yeah," I interrupted, "frantically stirring bubbling stone pots of fragrant Brazilian delicacies that are a little exotic, but still fall within the touristy categories of chicken, fish, or vegetarian. Meanwhile, Jose could regale the people with his never-ending stories."

"I'm a like this idea," Jose chimed in. "I give the peeps *cachaça*."

Mic responded, "Yeah, Jose, people love Brazilian rum! You could serve it to them in your hollowed-out gourd spoon."

"The tourists would love the idea of an industrious 11-year-old son being involved in the family farm," Jim said. "While dinner's cooking, Matheus could drive the tractor down to the corral while Jose and the guests sit in the spotless trailer behind him. Newborn calves would just *happen* to be there, and it would also just *happen* to be milking time."

Jose said, "I make cheese for the peeps and say, 'Friends. Come closer. I just make some fresh cheese with my cow milk. Try!'"

"Don't forget!" Ehris reminded everyone. "We need after-dinner entertainment starring Jose, Isabela, Matheus, and Fatima. Fatima could be handing out some kind of goody as Jose strums his guitar, Isabela sings, and Matheus plays the accordion."

I could picture the entire evening. The tourists would leave happy, a little drunk, and content, knowing they had experienced a night with an authentic Brazilian farm family and had the chance to give them some money to help them out. At the end of the night, Jose, wearing Adidas shorts, would plop down upstairs on his leather couch from Costco and flip through seven hundred channels on the flat screen TV they'd had shipped from the United States. Isabela would surf the Internet and bid on eBay items.

In the middle of the night, something happened to Jim. At about two A.M. he began pacing around, sweating and crying. This was totally unlike Jim, and I was freaking out. He was so worked up he wasn't even able to tell me what was going on. This was a guy who, every night, put his head on the pillow and actually told himself, *okay, body, it's time to go to sleep now,* while I tossed and turned and tried to get my brain to turn off. I was finally able to establish that he was tormented about leaving Jose's house in the morning. We had found a place where we wanted to be. Jose was like a brother, and none of us wanted to go back to life in Connecticut.

In the morning, both Jose and Jim cried and hugged. Jose walked us to the security checkpoint at the airport and kissed us all goodbye. As we prepared to head through security, I turned around and saw Jose standing there, sobbing. That image of Jose weeping is one I'll never forget. It's hard to say goodbye at any time or place. It's harder still to say it when a continent will soon separate you from the place you want to be. I stopped walking and turned my head, looking through the sliding-glass doors for a final wave. I can still picture the pale yellow shirt he was wearing. It's been said we are led to those who help us most to grow, and that people come into our lives for a reason. Maybe you learn that with every goodbye.

After many more trips to Brazil, we made the decision to move to Ponte Nova, which means *New Bridge* in Portuguese, the language of Brazil. The owner of the *hotel fazenda* didn't want to sell, but we decided we would run a dairy farm and open an English school.

Jose always reminded Jim, "Jeem, I do for you like you do for me," promising to repay Jim's kindness as he searched for a farm and helped build our herd of dairy cows, which lived on his enormous *fazenda* until we were ready to make our move. It took four years to prepare as we dreamed of our future.

CHAPTER FOURTEEN

Velya

"I can handle Daddy," my mother always insisted.

Everyone in the family was well aware of my father's verbal abuse, but pussyfooted around him at my mother's directive to keep the peace and not rock the boat.

Three weeks after we returned from our first trip to Brazil, my mother had a knee replacement. In the hospital, she was delirious and hallucinating. Giggling, she remarked that Jim, when he visited, had red lights twinkling all around his head.

"Veal, can I go downstairs and get you a cup of coffee?" she asked, though tethered to the bed with IV tubes, beeping machinery, and a catheter. Conspiratorially, she told me, "I wrote my name in clam shells under a boardwalk so people would know I had been there. Been there and done my best."

"It's the goddamn Ultracet!" my father hollered in the waiting room.

"What the heck are you talking about?" I asked, raising my eyebrows.

"She's been on the goddamn stuff for two and a half years," he said angrily. "They won't fill the prescription anymore at Ridgefield CVS. I have to get it at the Danbury CVS. She's addicted!"

"You mean Ultracet, the narcotic?" I asked, trying to understand. "Why is she taking Ultracet?"

"She started taking it after her hip replacement, and that fuckin' new Indian doctor of hers keeps refilling the prescription," he snarled. I thought, *but aren't you the one picking up the prescription and giving her the pills?*

I stayed with my mother round the clock, and she literally did not close her eyes for three days. She constantly reached in front of her for things that weren't there, keeping her hands in tight fists with her thumbs tucked in, which she had been doing for a year. As I sat alone in the hospital room, I pieced together that my mother was going through withdrawal.

"Mom, what's the deal with the Ultracet?" I probed during one of her lucid moments.

"I can't live with Daddy unless one of us is tranquilized," she said weakly. "You know he's not on Librax anymore." When our Filipino doctor retired, my father's new physician had convinced him to get off the medication. Ever since, he had become more explosive, impulsive, and mean. I guess my mother had been anesthetizing herself in order to numb her situation.

On the third morning of her withdrawal, my father launched into one of his raging tirades at an overworked hospital aide, who had been very kind to my confused mother. He bellowed, "Jesus Christ, what the fuck is wrong with you? Can't you see my wife needs help? Get in the room and take care of her, you goddamn bitch!"

As he screamed and swore at this Colombian woman, something in me snapped. *If you watch how a man treats people he considers little, you'll see how he treats you, if you let him,* I thought.

"Mommy doesn't need to hear this. Take it out in the hall!" I hissed, as we moved to the door. "Who do you think is still going to be in this hospital room when you go home tonight? What kind of care do you think she's going to get if the nurses think her husband is a nut job?"

"A nut job?!" my father roared.

"You're acting like an idiot and yelling at everyone like you always do, and then you leave the mess for someone else to clean up," I accused as we returned to the hospital room. I knew full well it would be my responsibility to apologize to the aide on my father's behalf.

Moments later, Jordan arrived. The next 45 minutes were probably the most bizarre of my life. My mother, who had barely uttered a coherent sentence in three days, spoke to my father as Jordan and I listened.

She told him, gently but firmly, "For the entire fifty-nine years of our marriage, I've walked on eggshells around you. We've *all* walked on eggshells around you. Whatever time I have left, I just want peace. I love you very much, but if you don't change, next time I'm not coming back."

Surprisingly, my father didn't storm out; he remained in the hospital room throughout her entire talk, and didn't shout her down. My mother told him she had never, in their entire marriage, been able to have a discussion with him. Amazingly—and this is truly amazing if you have any experience with daily life in a hospital—no one else entered the room for the entire 45 minutes. It was as I were looking through one of those one-way mirrors at some breakthrough moment in a counseling session, and my mother was both the counselor and the counselee.

There's no point in going over all that was said, except

she repeated over and over, "I just want peace." My father wandered around the room, stared out the window, and ultimately sat beside her with his elbows on the hospital bed, weeping and insisting things would change. "Just give me a chance to show you what kind of man I can be," he begged her. "Please don't leave me."

I didn't say anything at the time, but I noticed as soon as my mother finished talking to my father, she unclenched her fists. The next day, when Jim and I visited her at the hospital, her hands were open and still.

CHAPTER FIFTEEN

Ehris

After Nazey's knee replacement and Ultracet withdrawal, my mom quit her teaching job to take care of her. I knew how difficult the situation was, and wanted to help. I left Shepaug High School and started online school, with the plan of finishing my last three years of high school at *Escola Nossa Senhora Auxiliadora* in Ponte Nova. For a year and a half, my mom and I went to Ridgefield every day, often sleeping over.

When we got to my grandparents' house every morning, it was pretty clear from her slurred speech, spaciness, and concentration problems that Nazey had been given Xanax, her new sedative of choice to cope with my grandfather. We begged him not to give her tranquilizers, but he countered, "She's a lunatic without the drugs." By mid-morning, we'd have Nazey bathed, dressed, fed, and semi-coherent. Once, when my grandfather didn't realize I was in the house, I watched him sweep a whole stack of Nazey's crossword puzzle books off the coffee table and yell, "It's a goddamn shit house around here!" He barked at her, "You have dementia! You can't even *do* a fucking crossword puzzle!" I didn't tell my mom. I didn't want her heart to hurt any more than it already did.

It was clear that after Nazey's talk with him in the hospital, my grandfather hadn't become a better man. Nothing my mom and I were doing was fixing anything, but we hoped that once Nazey was back on her feet, she would finally stand up to him.

During the day, we would accompany my grandparents to all doctor's appointments, staying with Nazey while my grandfather swam at the Ridgefield Rec Center and did laundry at the laundromat (since septic tank failure was his phobia). We took Nazey to the movies, shopping, to the library, or out to lunch. My mom often cooked dinners at our house and brought them to Ridgefield. By the time we left in the late afternoon, Nazey would be cheerful. The frustrating, draining pattern would repeat every morning.

Velya

I turned 50 that year. I began to have a desire to get away, to have more time alone to figure out who I was, where I was, and what I wanted to do. Some may call this a mid-life crisis, but it wasn't—it was more like my quest for a self that was separate from my roles as daughter, sister, mother, and wife. When I began untangling years of emotional knots, I felt I was finally beginning to own my own skin after years of paying rent.

One of the knots I tried to unsnarl involved my only regret in life. When Mic and Ehris were very little, the three of us went to my parents' house for the day. The kids were lying on the living room floor watching *Sesame Street*. I was in the dining room with my father, who wanted to show me something from *The News-Times*, which he couldn't find. He started throwing stuff around the room, and I knew what was coming next.

"Where's the goddamn paper?!" he bellowed, and my mother came trotting. She started frantically searching, trying to calm him down. He pounded the dining room table and yelled, "Jesus fucking Christ! Can't you leave the goddamn newspaper where I put it?"

Normally, I would have helped my mother find the paper to de-escalate the situation. I was good at that. I had learned the art of abatement from a master. But that day was different.

"Oh, my god!" I exclaimed. Glancing into the living room, I begged, "Will you *please* stop? I heard enough of this while I was growing up. I don't need my own kids to hear it all, too!"

Like an erupting volcano, he spewed, "Who the hell do you think you're talking to? Get out of my house!"

I turned to my alarmed mother and asked, "Mom, do you want me to leave?" She shook her head as he slammed out the front door. I was shaken, but didn't regret what I had said, and told my mother exactly that. We hung out with my mom for a few more hours before I strapped the kids into their car seats and headed home.

The next morning, my father called me, which he never did, and said stiffly, "Your mother told me about all the stress you're under, and I accept your apology."

Stress I was under? Apology? What the heck was he talking about? And then I figured it out. My mother had gone into full-blown damage control and concocted an apology to assuage the situation. And here's the part that eats away at me, the part I wish I could do over: I went along with it. I went along with it because she had done a masterful job of brainwashing me about not cracking those damn eggshells—about avoiding them at all costs, no matter what you had to give up in return. I could have changed the whole dynamic of the relationship if I had told the truth. I have to live with that. I had already become a people-pleaser, and this incident only strengthened my father's sick power in the family.

At the insistence of my mother, I had always tiptoed around my father. I hadn't rocked the boat, hadn't made any waves. I had followed her rules. If only I could have known that bullies back down when they're confronted. This concocted apology created the first crack in my relationship with my mother.

At age 50, I began to feel like the happy girl I had been at Ridgebury Elementary School; the bossy little tomboy who was always up a tree or down a hole, a water sprite when it came to swimming, queen of turtle hunting and bringing home stray animals. Cheerleading never made much sense to me, and I never dressed up like a princess on Halloween. The tween years are tricky ages in the life of a tomboy, however, and eventually, I wasn't able to make my sprouting breasts disappear, no matter how baggy my T-shirts were. That first little spot of blood in my white cotton underwear (they were *not* panties), embarrassment over puberty, shaving, plucking, being pretty on the outside, learning to filter—they all brought about the death of the bossy little tomboy. The beginnings of menopause brought her back to life.

Self-knowledge and self-confidence were the true gifts of my menopause. Of course, hot flashes sucked, but in a way,

I felt as if they were setting my brain on fire and creating an inner glow. Sometimes, I had so many creative ideas I felt as if I held a volcanic energy within me, and hot lava needed to flow. I finally understood Margaret Mead's famous quote: "The most powerful force in the world is a menopausal woman with zest."

My earliest memory of anything to do with menopause was my mother having a hysterectomy in her early 40s. She must have experienced menopausal symptoms. Nothing, absolutely nothing was talked about—how having the hysterectomy made her feel, what symptoms she was experiencing, or how she was coping. It was a taboo subject. When our nosy neighbor, Mrs. Roth, asked six-year-old Jordan why our mother was in the hospital, he responded, "She has overlapping ovaries."

People leave odd little memories of themselves behind. It's funny how you don't remember all the boring details leading up to the memory. It's like *pow*, you're instantly in your playclothes with your friends, fascinated by the fact that your mom has done something magical to the canister vacuum. Instead of it being on "suck" mode, it's on "blow" mode. Suddenly, she's blowing up balloons with the vacuum and knotting them. Enormous balloons. Not the round kind, but the hotdog shaped ones. You're sword fighting with them and batting them all over the cathedral ceiling living room, not letting them hit the oval braided rug. And then the memory just stops, as memories do.

It wasn't until I was a grown-up that I realized the balloons had been condoms. That's when it all gets sort of weird. Piecing things together, I'm thinking this was after her hysterectomy. We were allowed to wave up at her room from the Danbury Hospital parking lot, but didn't really know the mysterious reason she was there. Is it weird because the balloons are tangible proof that my parents had a sex life? My mother's hysterectomy forced her into early menopause. Was she okay with that? Was the balloon thing akin to bra burning? Was she now free of the need for contraceptives? Or did she just go a little bonkers on that rainy afternoon in the living room? When our friends became grown-ups, did they look back and realize we had been sword fighting with condoms? Do they even remember it at all?

After 18 months, Ehris and I weaned my mother off Xanax and arranged for a live-in caregiver. I had dropped everything to take care of my mother and help my father. I wanted to move forward in my life, but I still had one foot on the brake. Maybe it had something to do with turning 50, but it also had something to do with Ehris and the example I wanted to set. It's okay to be a devoted caregiver, but not when you're sacrificing yourself for people who aren't even trying to help themselves. After decades of dutiful-daughter service to my parents, I took my foot off the brake and typed "Brazil" into my GPS.

CHAPTER SIXTEEN

Ehris

The day we cleaned out the attic was the first time I ever saw my dad cry. I didn't realize how sad it had all gotten until we started digging through the past. My mom, dad, and I had held it together while we were sorting through the attic. We were getting ready to put our house on the market. Stored in the attic, certain items had been "out of sight, out of mind." It wasn't until we took a break and sat on the porch swing that all three of us began to cry. There were too many sweet memories—some so sad, they couldn't be washed away by tears.

The Rubbermaid bin of Barbies. Mic and I had named all of them, and wrote and filmed countless Barbie movies. The plots always included sinister Dick Blick kidnapping blonde, wholesome Amy Sylvester.

The two wooden stables my dad had built for us. Every plastic horse had its own hand-labeled stall, where it returned each night after trail rides under the coffee table, up the spiral staircase, and around the dog bowls. Mic's favorite horse was a lively Appaloosa he named Stardancer.

The Cozy Coupe, which Mic and I called the "Cat Food Express." With a jump rope, we would tie a red metal wagon to the back of the Cozy Coupe. When the wagon was filled with cat food cans, Mic would lift me into the open trunk and hop in the driver's seat. We would drive all over the house, making very important cat food deliveries.

The 4-H Poultry Showmanship ribbons. On lazy summer days, my mom would sit outside on our porch swing with Mic and quiz him on the 100 possible showmanship questions he might be required to answer at the annual 4-H fair. I think we knew all the answers to the questions just as well as he did: What is the bleaching order of a chicken? At what temperature does a rooster's comb freeze? What is the purpose of the preen gland? Why do we measure the flexibility of the pubic bone?

During showmanship, Mic would have to demonstrate different holds, locate the sternum, keel, and axial feathers, and then hold the chicken backward and eye-level with the judges, and push aside the feathers and display the vent (where the egg comes out), all while wearing white pants. Do you know how hard it was for my mom to find white pants for a six-foot-tall, 13-year-old boy without having to spend a lot of money on them, because obviously he wasn't going to wear them in real life? After weeks of searching, she finally found an almost-okay pair at Goodwill. They were kind of cream-colored, but with a little bleaching, she hoped they could work. My dad came home one day with a bottle of leftover bleach he'd needed for a power-washing job. We put the pants in a full bucket of bleach, and put the bucket in the bathtub overnight. The bleach fumes were blinding the next morning, but when I looked in the bucket, the pants looked really white. We all assembled in the bathroom for the unveiling. Mic plunged his hand into the bucket and pulled out a wad of wet, shredded napkins. His pants had disintegrated in the bleach, leaving only the zipper and the metal button tab. My dad put on his Walmart reading glasses to examine the bleach bottle label. It was actually contractor bleach, and two tablespoons were meant to be diluted with one gallon of water. We laughed all the way back to Goodwill.

There had always been a lot of laughing in our house. That ended when Mic was in high school.

Velya

I remember Jim coming home from work and snatching up baby Ehris, who would hold out her arms like an airplane as they ran around the house chasing a shrieking Mic. Jim called, "I'm gonna get that boy, I'm gonna get that boy!" Mic on the kitchen counter, sitting cross-legged in navy blue slipper socks, licking birthday-cake beaters while Ehris methodically counted 83 pieces of ziti with her toddler fingers. "Yup, Ehris. I need exactly 83 pieces for this special recipe for Daddy."

Even though we planned to take the height chart with us to Brazil, there were two things we couldn't take, but I thought of them every time I saw a daffodil. As weird as it may sound, I couldn't bear to throw away my babies' umbilical cords when they fell off. I couldn't picture something so life-giving just winding up in a garbage can. That's why I planted Mic's umbilical cord in front of the house down by the daffodils, and when it was Ehris's turn, Mic solemnly helped me plant hers.

I only have to close my eyes to remember the summer day when Jim, Mic, and Ehris built the gabled playhouse with gingerbread trim. Ehris was clad in only red plaid sneakers, a diaper, and a canvas tool belt. Jim bravely held the nails as a two- and four-year-old whacked his fingers more times than they whacked the nails. The Sunday morning when we were all wrestling on our bed. Mic's white sock got caught in Jim's big toe toenail, and in a flash, it pulled out the entire toenail by the roots. Jim assured a tearful Mic it was okay—it didn't hurt a bit. And under the incredible nine tons of cement and fieldstone Jim had labored over, I knew exactly where in our front walk Mic and Ehris had buried Stonyfield yogurt-container time capsules filled with their treasured possessions and private messages.

Mic ruined these memories. Life imploded when he turned 16, and the years of him hating Connecticut—and us—began. To this day, I don't know what triggered it all. I don't know if he even does. Good parenting, in large part, consists of creating positive memories for your children. We had given Mic and Ehris freedom at an early age because they had earned our trust. Through the 4-H international exchange program, we'd let them test their wings in places like Estonia, Scotland, and South Korea. Had giving Mic his independence created this mess? We had been four people who sincerely cared about each other. There had always been a deep connection, trust, and respect. It's the things that blindside you that hurt the most.

Sometimes, I think there's something wrong with me, because I only remember fragments of those awful years. There are things you forget, like passwords and locker combinations—and there are things you can't forget that you wish you could. One memory I wish I *could* erase took place in our living room. Mic was sitting on our velvet Victorian settee when he calmly declared to Jim, "I hate you. I even hate the way you chew," as if he were an emotionless Supreme Court justice handing down a final ruling. I still can't look at that piece of furniture without remembering the broken look on Jim's face. That was when he stopped talking to Mic. I don't know if Mic ever apologized to Jim, but I don't think it would have mattered. Jim is a man of action, not words. Mic said all kinds of things without ever opening his mouth.

Perhaps to another family, a Facebook profile that included "I hate my parents" wouldn't be such a big deal. People have clucked at me, "Oh, that's just kids going through their teen years. Every kid does that." In our family, however, this was akin to a fast stab wound to the heart. When someone stabs you, the pain you feel isn't your fault. When Jordan saw Mic's declaration, he posted, "I won't tolerate you talking about my sister and brother-in-law this way. Your parents gave you an idyllic childhood." After that, Jordan lost respect for Mic. Even today, Jordan has an underlying disdain for him. There is great truth in my mother's index card: "You are the master of the unspoken word; once it leaves your lips, you are its slave forever."

I was stunned when Jim, who never expressed or discussed his feelings, arranged for all four of us to go to family counseling. Mic would target one victim at a time. He would try to pit the three of us against each other, and knew each of our Achilles heels. In a family counseling session, he revealed his arrogant contempt for Jim when he compared Jim to Boxer, the cart-horse from George Orwell's *Animal Farm*. Mic viewed Boxer as ignorant, dimwitted, and unable to think for himself. To me, Boxer's incredible strength, dedication, hard work, loyalty, protection of the other animals, and ability to keep the farm together made him the most beloved character of the novel. During another session, we were discussing Mic's lying. Without our permission or knowledge, he had driven three hours to Albany, New York to visit a guy he had met online. Mic was 16; the guy was 26. The counselor, trying to get Mic to understand our concern, asked, "Velya and Jim, can you explain to Mic why you were so upset about this incident?"

Jim nodded and said seriously, "Mic, it doesn't matter to us if you were meeting a man or a woman. You know we don't care about that. But this person was a stranger, ten years older than you."

"Mic," I continued. "What could a twenty-six-year-old man possibly have in common with a sixteen-year-old boy? Why would he be interested in you? Daddy and I are worried about your safety."

Mic smirked, "You had no idea what I was doing when I was in Estonia. I don't want to have to answer to anybody. I don't want any rules."

Three of us were willing to put in the work, but counseling is only effective if everyone involved admits there's a problem. The months of counseling fizzled out when we realized it was going nowhere. At what would be our final session, the counselor chirped, "Velya, what kind of animal are you? What kind of animal is Jim?" We had to take turns and go around the room and explain why I thought I was a horse, Jim thought Ehris was a dolphin, Ehris thought Mic was a cobra, and Mic thought I was a Komodo dragon. Given the fact that our kid was engaging in risky behaviors and our family was falling apart, this seemed pretty unproductive.

Mic begged us to let him spend his senior year of high school in Paraguay through the American Field Service program. While he was gone, we didn't exchange newsy letters, and we didn't mail him chocolate-chip-cookie care packages. Frankly and honestly, we didn't talk about him at all. Years later, Mic said, "I just want to thank you guys so much for the gift of letting me go to Paraguay."

"It wasn't a gift, Mic," I said dully. "None of us could stand being around you. We sent you there because it hurt too much to have you here."

During those lousy, apocalyptic years, forging a fake smile safeguarded my emotions. A smile is powerful camouflage. It's possible to hide sorrow, pain, and heartache behind a smile, but eyes don't lie. If anyone had taken the time to look into my eyes, they would have seen it. There was a hole in my heart from the damage Mic had inflicted.

After Mic came back from Paraguay, nothing had changed. Jim still wasn't speaking to him, which only added to the horrible atmosphere in our once-loving home. The magic of nightly family dinner had always been a shared connection—our favorite time of the day. During the crappy years, there were many nights I would've liked to hit Jim in the head with the pork chops and smear mashed potatoes all over Mic's face. The silent treatment had always been Jim's passive-aggressive way of dealing with problems. Every time it happened, those childhood memories of my father's silent treatments resurfaced: the dread and tension, the wishing he would just yell at us rather than ignore us.

When prisoners are punished, guards isolate them, because being isolated is one of the harshest punishments there is, other than physical abuse. Usually, Jim's episodes lasted a few days until I'd rescue and cajole him out of his funk, just so peace could be restored in the family. Jim was hurt and angry, but refused to talk about what was bothering him. He wouldn't do the work of expressing his feelings and moving toward a solution. Instead, he attempted to ignore Mic through protracted silence. While Mic was his target, Ehris and I were the casualties.

Ehris and I tried, unsuccessfully, to jolly Jim out of his silence. One day, six months into the mute punishment, it ended as suddenly as it had begun. The four of us were watching a movie, *P.S. I Love You*, in our living room. The premise was that Holly, a young widow, discovers that her late husband, Gerry, has left her ten notes intended to help ease her grief and start a new life. Holly's mother and friends begin to worry that Gerry's letters are keeping Holly tied to the past, but in fact, each letter is pushing her further into a new future. With Gerry's words as her guide, Holly embarks upon a journey of rediscovery in a story about marriage, friendship, and how a love so strong can turn the finality of death into a new beginning for life.

When Holly opened the fourth letter from Gerry, Jim's chest started heaving. He sniffled and wiped his eyes continuously for the rest of the film. I glanced at Ehris, raising my eyebrows as if to ask, "What's going on? Why is he crying?" While the letter was heartfelt, I didn't see any connection between it and Jim's life. It said, "You don't need my belongings to remember me by, you don't need to keep them as proof that I existed or still exist in your mind." Ehris responded with a shrug of her shoulders and raised her eyebrows back at me. She and I averted our gaze, pretending not to notice Jim's sobbing, just like when someone sitting next to you farts, and you pretend you don't notice so they don't feel bad. When the movie ended, the silent treatment ended.

Nothing was discussed. It was just over—but it wasn't really over. Every time Jim had ended a silent treatment episode, my relief that it was over was greater than my anger at his refusal to talk about what had triggered it. Looking back on it with tremendous guilt, I don't know how I allowed any of this to happen, but it takes a lot of years to see patterns. Jim grew up in a family that didn't talk about anything, let alone feelings. I grew up brainwashed about not rocking the boat. The combination was the perfect recipe for sweeping conflict under the rug.

Years later, I learned that when *P.S. I Love You* and the silent treatment ended, Mic, overjoyed, had gone to the upstairs of our barn and shared his happiness through a phone call to a family friend. While I don't condone the way Jim handled the situation, Mic never treated him with disrespect again. Well-timed silence can carry more power than speech. This tough love made an impact on Mic, but it wasn't fair to Ehris or me. Caught in the crossfire, our relationship changed from mother and child to allies in a gloomy existence.

There were wonderful memories of Mic and my parents in every corner of our Bridgewater house, but it hurt too much to live amongst them. I had to stop remembering, so I packed away the family photo albums and home videos. They're in a safe place, but I'm still not brave enough to open up the bubble wrap and pain. Our house was no longer a home. I learned that if you decide to leave a place where you have lived and loved—where memories are buried even deeper than Stonyfield time capsules—leave it as fast as you can. Just treat it like a Band-Aid. Don't pull up a corner a little at a time. Rip it off, and give the wound some air. Let the tougher skin form. And know that no matter how fast you yank the Band-Aid off, it will always leave a sticky adhesive residue behind, an outline of what used to be, on your skin.

PART TWO

"Don't you find it odd," she continued, "that when you're a kid, everyone, all the world, encourages you to follow your dreams. But when you're older, somehow they act offended if you even try."

—ETHAN HAWKE,
The Hottest State

CHAPTER SEVENTEEN

Velya

"Why can't you just be like everyone else and move to Florida?" our accountant implored. He tapped his mechanical pencil and studied me as if I were an intrepid, or possibly insane, bonnet-topped pioneer woman about to join a wagon train for parts unknown. I could picture a CAT scan of his brain at that exact moment, short-circuiting as it computed, *they are out of their minds!*

"We're not having a reckless midlife crisis," I explained. "We just want to try something new."

"But *Brazil?*" he groaned. "Don't they have anacondas there? And piranhas? Do any of you even know how to speak Spanish?" Massaging his temples, he continued, "It means you'll have to file a Form 2555, Form 1116, and a F-I-N-C-114."

To our accountant, pulling off our move from Bridgewater, Connecticut to Ponte Nova, Brazil was as unlikely as the Donner party making it through the snowy Sierra Nevadas without cannibalizing each other.

In his desire to get as far away from Connecticut as he could, Mic had applied for acceptance to the Heritage Program at the University of Puerto Rico, which was intended for children of Puerto Rican immigrants to rediscover their roots. Although he didn't have one drop of Puerto Rican blood, his essay about his fictional Puerto Rican ancestry was such a convincingly persuasive lie that he was accepted. Since the situation with him had improved a little, he would stay with us in Ponte Nova at summer break.

As we set sail into the sea of uncertainty, our course didn't make sense to family or friends. People weighed in with their life rules and fears, but we decided *to eeny, meeny, miney,* go.

"You're moving to Brazil?" I was asked in the dog food aisle at Stop & Shop.

"Yes."

"Are you Brazilian?" I was asked at the hair salon.

"No."

"Your husband is Brazilian?" I was asked at the Mobil station.

"No."

"Do you have family in Brazil?" I was asked at the library.

"No."

In the post office parking lot, the mother of one of my former students patted my arm and revealed, "Oh, we were talking about all of you at dinner last night. You're so brave to just pick up and move to a foreign country. Ehris must be psyched to do her last two years of high school there. I'd never have the courage!" I heard this wherever I went, but it never felt that way to any of us. There was a whole new continent out there, and we were excited, but never scared.

I generally responded, "We just want to try something new. There's nothing mysterious about it. We just want to make a change."

Ehris

For months, Jose searched for farms for us. He called and described each one. Sometimes, when he emailed photos, I imagined myself galloping around on a friendly horse with a silky mane, stopping to knock coconuts from palm trees and hopping off to eat bananas in the shade of a bamboo grove. We became more and more frustrated each time a potential farm purchase fell through.

We already had a golf cart, but decided to buy a new one to use at our Brazilian farm, and give the one we already had to Jose as a thank-you gift for everything he was doing for us. Since I always got stuck with any kind of job that involved a computer, I did some research to find out which model would be the best for driving around in the infamously gloppy mud of Brazil, carrying bags of feed, and transporting us and our guests. At Tractor Supply, we found one that would be perfect for our needs. It was forest green and had space in the back for storage.

Our house was on the market, and there were many days when we felt like it would never sell, and we'd never be able to start our new adventure in Brazil. On discouraging days like this, we'd drive over to Tractor Supply and visit our future golf cart. My mom, dad, and I would sit in the front seat of the parked golf cart and pretend to be driving in Brazil. We would say things like, "Jeem, don't hit that *tatu* in the middle of the road!" And we would wave and greet our future neighbors by exclaiming, "*Oi, vizinho!*" We were pathetic, and we knew it.

We eventually did buy the forest green golf cart, and named it "Joe Cats" after our insurance agent (that really was his name). Joe once told us that he admired our courage to pack up and go to Brazil. He said that he was such a creature of habit that he never ventured past the Lake Lillinonah bridge into neighboring Brookfield. Soon, "Joe Cats" would be having the adventure of a lifetime!

All of our energies were focused on Brazil. We worked for, planned for, took Portuguese lessons for, and dreamed of our new lives.

CHAPTER EIGHTEEN

Ehris

S ome Americans who hear our story think that we foolishly and impulsively just packed up and moved to Brazil on a whim. We had actually visited Brazil many times, and took all the necessary steps to start new lives on a new continent.

On one of our trips to Ponte Nova, we realized we'd have to buy a car, and it would be easier to do it before the big move. Along with our herd of cows (we now had 200), the car would live at Jose's farm until we were ready.

My dad wavered a million times between buying a truck, a used small car, a used big car, a diesel, or a flex-fuel. In Brazil, there are lots of colorful old VW Bugs with the silver handle on the hood. At a used car lot in Ponte Nova, we looked at a 1983 yellow VW for $19,000 *real* (about $9,500 United States dollars). Things like houses and food are cheaper in Brazil, but clothes and cars are much more expensive than in the United States. This car seemed like it was in pretty good shape, and it was the older style beetle, not that new kind with the glass bud vase in the front. One of the guys who worked there told us that we could go for a test drive. He was wearing tight black nylon pants and a black spandex T-shirt with the words "Scottish Knight" (in English) in large gold letters.

In Brazil, we saw lots of unsuspecting non-English speakers, from small children to old ladies, who had no idea that they were wearing swear words, racist and sexist terms, or phrases that didn't make sense on their t-shirts. A teenage boy hawking jackfruit wore a royal blue shirt proclaiming "Naughty Witch" in a spooky font. At the post office, the pale pink shirt on a frail woman with a dowager's hump declared her a "Savage Warrior."

Jose, who had driven us to the used car lot, said, "Jeem, you take this car to VW dealer. They tell you if it worth the money."

My mom and I climbed into the back seat. Actually, we slithered behind the tilted-forward front seats, and once we sat down, my head hit the ceiling. I sat at a diagonal, and couldn't see out the window because it was too low for my line of vision. My mom fit in just fine. My dad got into the driver's seat and looked like Paul Bunyan driving a Barbie car. Mic's knees hit the dashboard, and he got hair gel all over the roof upholstery.

My dad zipped past the mopeds and mule carts with his international driver's license in his back pocket (that sounds really official, but really, it was a paper booklet with his smiling photo stapled to the front, issued by AAA for $26.95). He somehow already knew where the Volkswagen dealership was, and pulled in. We all squeezed out the doors and walked into the garage. Since I had moved on to level three of our Portuguese class (while my parents were still struggling with basic introductions), I asked one of the mechanics if he could take a look at the car, and he pleasantly agreed. There was an uncomfortable metal bench inside where we sat and waited for over an hour. The mechanic finally reappeared, and told me the car was worth $9,000 *real* (about $2,800 United States dollars). We didn't want to spend a lot of money on a car, since we also planned to buy a truck, so getting an overpriced Volkswagen we couldn't even fit into was not a good idea.

During the hour on the metal bench, we'd discussed buying a used gray VW Gol we had seen in the dealership parking lot. When we went into the showroom, I wasn't sure if they were still in business. During this trip to Ponte Nova, it had rained nonstop for seven days, which caused the town's worst flooding in 100 years. In some areas, it looked like New Orleans after Hurricane Katrina. Bridges were totally washed out, sidewalks were destroyed, there were branches and trees all over the roads, and many people were stranded in their houses. In the VW showroom, there were watermarks on the walls, and it was obvious that the desks had been ruined, because they had makeshift plywood tables and mismatched chairs. There weren't even any cars in the showroom. A few moments later, a grinning salesman walked in and asked if we needed help. He had no idea what he was in for!

Luis, the salesman, noticed pretty quickly that we were not Brazilians. Because Luis only spoke Portuguese, all of my dad's car questions had to be translated through me. My dad had probably bought 34 cars in his lifetime, and knew what he was talking about. He asked in English, "What size is the engine? What's the rear-end ratio? Is it total flex or diesel? What's the compression ratio of the pistons?" Other Connecticut 15-year-olds were buying jeans at the mall with their mom's debit card, but here I was, negotiating on a car in Brazil. Even in English, I had no idea what my dad was talking about, but I had to translate all of this for Luis. My Portuguese/English dictionary didn't have words like crankshaft, valve covers, and timing belt, so I had to improvise.

Another thing that made it difficult was that my dad would start asking Luis a question in his limited "Portuguese," and Luis wouldn't understand, so my dad would finish the question in English. Then, I would have to decode what my dad was trying to say and explain it to bewildered Luis. In the United States, my parents make a good team when it comes to buying a car. They kind of reel the salesman in, and then play the "good cop, bad cop" game. But in Brazil, I had to be both cops. Luis was obviously already familiar with this tactic. My dad would tell me to tell Luis that the car was expensive. I translated, *"O carro e caro,"* which is a hard phrase to pronounce. Luis would argue that the car wasn't expensive, and I would agree with him, but then remember that I was supposed to be on my dad's side. Meanwhile, my dad would keep talking and not give me time to translate. Mic and my mom were just lounging in their chairs, relaxing, drinking water, going to the bathroom, and saying stuff like, "Wow! Look at the flood damage!" My mom admired a framed photo of Luis's kids and told him (in English) how cute they were and how much they looked like him, which interrupted my intense negotiation. We wanted the gray Gol, and had a secret discussion in English that Luis couldn't understand.

"Ehris," my dad said out of the corner of his mouth, "Let's try and get new tires thrown in."

"Okay, just tell me what you want me to say. I think he'll go for it," I answered slyly.

In a low voice (which was pointless, since Luis didn't know any English), my dad said, "He'll probably only go for two, and that's okay, but still, try for four. Tell him that we'll buy the car if he'll throw in four tires."

I translated for Luis that we wanted four new *pneus* put on the car. Do you realize what a stupid word *pneu* is when you say it aloud? It's not a silent "p" like in "pneumonia." You pronounce the "p" and then put your lips in a weird position to finish the word, which sounds like "neeeyww."

Luis said no, he couldn't put on any *pneus*. He went to talk to his boss to see what he could work out, the same routine as in the United States. He came back and said that his boss said they would give us one *pneu*.

My dad told me to try again, and try to trick him. I confirmed with Luis, "So, we'll buy the car, and you said you'll throw in four *pneus*, right?"

Luis looked at me like I was crazy. He said in Portuguese, "No, we said one *pneu*, remember?"

Playing dumb, I said, "Okay, when are you going to install the four *pneus*?"

Luis said in Portuguese, "Did you understand? I said one *pneu*."

I was trying not to laugh as I responded, "Three? You said three *pneus*?"

Luis gave up and told us that he would install two new *pneus* on our car, and we could pay for the other two. We were able to buy the car and temporarily register it. Luis said he would help us with the permanent registration once we returned to Brazil. Sometimes it pays not to speak the language and have your 15-year-old daughter do the negotiating.

We shook hands, and my dad joked, "Luis, you really *do* speak English!"

Luis looked puzzled when I translated. He said that he didn't speak our language at all.

My dad chuckled, "Yes, you do: salami, elephant, banana!" This had become my dad's favorite phrase. For the first time that afternoon, Luis understood what my dad was saying, and laughed. In Portuguese, those three words are pronounced almost the same way as we say them. I'm sure Luis went home that night with stories about the crazy Americans who bought the two-door gray VW Gol.

Velya

One of the reasons we bought a car before our actual move to Brazil was so we wouldn't be dependent on Jose to drive us around. Several months before that trip to Ponte Nova, Jose had called, saying accusingly, "Jeem, you try kill me!"

Shocked, Jim asked, "What?"

Jose continued, "Jeem, you know that *escada laranja* you sell me two years ago?"

"You mean that heavy ladder I warned you not to buy from me?" Jim clarified.

Jose chuckled, "Yes, that's the ladder I fall off! You try kill me!"

Jose had been up on the ladder trying to fix the phone line going to his house (they're always having trouble with phone reception in that part of rural Brazil). He started fiddling around with the wires on top of a tall telephone pole in the middle of the pasture. He didn't feel like moving the ladder, so he stretched his arm to jiggle a wire, and as he stretched, the ladder started to wobble. He fell 16 feet to the ground.

Somehow, he crawled to the house, where Isabela and three of their workers got him into the back of their Fiat and rushed to the Ponte Nova Emergency Room. Diagnosed with a bad bruise, he was sent home, but in the middle of the night, his legs became numb. They drove three and a half hours to the hospital in Belo Horizonte, where he underwent 15 hours of surgery because his back was broken and his vertebra was pushing on his spinal cord. He had to stay in the hospital for eight days. Isabela called us from the waiting room with the terrible news.

Initially, Jose couldn't feel his arm, and they thought that it might be paralyzed. Of course, we told Isabela that we would cancel our upcoming trip, but she protested, saying the best medicine for Jose would be to see Jim. A few days later, Jim was able to speak briefly with Jose. Jose told him that he was just so *"happ"* to be alive, he didn't care if he never had feeling in his arm again.

Since Jose's back was broken and he was in a thick plastic brace that looked like a turtle shell, Jim offered to plant an acre of *capim* that Jose needed in order to feed his cows.

In Brazil, they plant *capim*, which they grind and feed to cows during the dry season, just as we do with hay in the winter. It's like sugar cane, but can be harvested three to four times a year. If you take care of *capim* by fertilizing it, it will grow forever. You have to dig furrows, then place chopped-up hunks of something resembling green palm fronds into the trenches. There are no roots involved, and I can't think of anything in the United States that grows like this, except maybe forsythia. So, taking machetes and a Brazilian version of a hoe along with us, Jim, Mic, Ehris, and I took the mile-long, nearly vertical walk up to Jose's field.

At first, it wasn't so bad. It was a bit daunting to see how big an acre actually was, but I figured with all of us pitching in, we'd get the job done in about 45 minutes. Ten minutes in, I thought I was going to die of heat stroke.

Jim, the time-and-motion study expert, advised us in monotone, "You have to think of your body as a machine. Don't waste any motions. Don't think about anything. Just think about the job and getting it done. You are a machine."

We all headed to different sections of the area and began to cover up the pieces of *capim*, which had already been laid in the furrows, with dirt. As I write this, it certainly doesn't sound like a very difficult process but, as Mic said, "It was like death."

Actually, Ehris and I covered the *capim*. Jim and Mic were chopping the lengths into smaller pieces. There were hunks of junky weed roots tangled up in the dirt, and paranoid Ehris was constantly on the lookout for scorpions and snakes. Okay, perhaps she wasn't paranoid, but the *capim* did not have her full attention. I vowed there and then and that if necessary, I would sell all my worldly possessions once we got home and buy a tractor. This experience was something out of a Third World country. Oh, that's right—we *were* in a Third World country!

Jim's rationale was that he had wanted to see the entire *capim* process from start to finish in order to improve upon it on our future farm. Over and over, we raised the wooden-handled hoes as high as our shoulders and pulled dirt over the trenches. I had just seen that 1932 movie *I Am a Fugitive from a Chain Gang* with Paul Muni, and half-expected an African-American chain gang guy to start belting out a motivational spiritual like "Raise 'em high …"

I glanced over at Ehris, who was working very hard, but wasn't sweating. I was so sweaty that my eyebrow pencil was running into my eyes, which I knew because of the stinging, and my light pink racerback sports bra was soaked. Mic and I agreed that we would have paid twenty bucks for a Diet Coke (excuse me, in Brazil, it's *Coca Zero*).

Ehris looked as cool as a cucumber, which had me very concerned. Though I am prone to exaggeration, it was easily 105 degrees in that field, and any normal person would have been drenched in sweat. I told Ehris that she had to climb back down the mountain and sit under a tree. Being Ehris, she argued with me, because she felt bad that the three of us were stuck with the job.

Since we had thought this was going to be a quick planting, we hadn't brought any water or hats, and the sun blazed. I was doing a fraction of the work of Mic and Jim. About two hours into the project, it began to rain, thank goodness, and cooled us off a bit. Mic and I started giving each other sweaty pep talks when we met at the end of a row.

"Only twenty-five more rows, Mic," I gasped.

"You can do it, Mommy," he encouraged. "Hang in there. Think about that *Coca Zero!*"

Finally, all the *capim* was covered. Jim was content, and we headed back down to find Ehris. Mic's hands were covered with already-popped bloody blisters. He and I picked mangoes as we hobbled down the hill. Mic and I collapsed into a shallow stream and dramatically drank water on our hands and knees.

Mic lifted his head like a thirsty horse and sighed happily, "This is the best water I've ever tasted."

"You're not kidding. I don't even care what kind of microscopic stuff is swimming around in here," I added.

That night, we experienced our first Brazilian rodeo, which is much different from rodeos in the United States. The traditional American rodeo begins when a glitzy cowgirl rides around waving the American flag as Lee Greenwood's "God Bless the U.S.A." blares over the PA system. The crowd gets all fired up at the line, "…and I'm proud to be an American, where at least I know I'm free."

A Brazilian rodeo isn't necessarily PBR-sanctioned, but it's much more fun. The food stalls offer *churrasco*, rice and beans, and Skol or Brahma beer. The women get very dressed up in pointy-toed stiletto cowboy boots and low-rise jeans, while the men wear their dress-up cowboy boots and fanciest belts with big silver buckles. Their collared, long-sleeved cowboy shirts with snaps are tucked neatly into their carefully ironed jeans. These aren't flannel shirts like the Marlboro man. They're cotton, usually black and red, with symmetrical designs and embroidery. It would be rare to find an American guy wearing one of these shirts. Samba and country music plays as the fans mingle and grab random partners for an impromptu dance. Although there's a lot of beer drinking going on, the crowd isn't dangerous or destructive.

As the crowd takes their seats, the announcer screams into the microphone in Portuguese. After some thank-yous to sponsors, an honored person gets to bring out a three-foot-tall Virgin Mary in a glass box. The Virgin Mary is paraded around, held up for the crowd to see. The cowboys all line up and take a knee in the dirt ring for *"A Oração do Cowboy"*

(The Cowboy Prayer). They remove their hats and hold them over their hearts. This prayer goes on for at least ten minutes as the announcer asks God to protect the cowboys from harm. The announcer concludes the prayer with an "*Amém.*"

Sometimes, the audience gets a real treat. At this rodeo, we watched one of the clowns doing something with what looked like a big bag of powdered chalk in the center of the ring. After they brought out the provocatively-dressed Rodeo Queen for her photo ops, the lights were turned off and someone brought out a flaming torch—the kind waved by angry mobs of villagers in *Frankenstein* movies. They held the torch to the ground, and the powdered chalk ignited into a flaming cross. In Portuguese, the crowd gasped, "*Ooh, aah!*"

CHAPTER NINETEEN

Ehris

If you've ever sold a house (which is what we had to do before we could move to Brazil), you know how frustrating it is. It's kind of like living in limbo because you have to pretend you don't live there, but you really do. Everything needs to be kept neat and tidy at all times, since you never know when you're going to have a showing. Getting ready for one includes emptying all the garbage cans, lighting the non-offensively scented "Clean Linen" Yankee Candles, carrying the 75-pound metal dog kennel outside, down the stairs, and into the creepy, dark, dirt-floor basement, Swiffer-ing the kitchen tile floor while Cairn terrier Chauncey and Great Dane Sylvia are pacing and panting because they know they're going for a ride in the car, turning on the right lamps to "set the mood," putting out the Lindt truffles to lure the prospective buyers, and Windex-ing nose prints off the French doors.

When my parents were building one of their many additions, they decided to include a spiral staircase in the dining room. The center supporting pipe was hollow, and had a removable wooden decoration on top. Over the years, Mic and I dropped many things down the pipe, including Barbies with bad haircuts, plastic dinosaurs, and secret notes.

My mom, dad, and I were getting a little crazy in anticipation of starting our new lives. One day, my mom shrieked,
"Oh, my god! I have the best idea!" She found a bag of mixed
nuts in the kitchen cabinet and took out three Brazil nuts.
"Everybody, pick a nut and write some motivational stuff on
it," she ordered. With black Sharpie markers, we each drew
inspirational pictures and messages on the shells. My dad
drew a stick-figure horse. My mom wrote *Vender nossa casa!*
which meant *Sell our house!* on one side of the nut, and drew
a map of Brazil on the other. I drew myself milking *Formiga*.
Drawing on a bumpy Brazil nut isn't easy. When our drawings
were complete, we assembled at the top of the spiral staircase
and ceremoniously removed the wooden cover. At the exact
same moment, we dropped the Brazil nuts down the pipe,
and while they clattered to the bottom, we chanted stuff like,
"Oi, vizinho!" (Hey, neighbor!) and *"A senhora sabe onde fica o
hotel?"* (Ma'am, do you know where the hotel is?). These were
the only two phrases my dad could ever remember from his
"Learn Portuguese: Volume I" CD.

Finally, Jose found us the perfect farm. "Jeem, you no
believe!" he said excitedly over the phone. "I find for you a
fazenda with papaya trees, a *heever* (river), room for the cows,
and a house." He said that when we were ready, he would
have the *corral* built and our herd of 200 cows shipped over
from his farm. Surprisingly, the next day, we had an offer on
our Bridgewater house, which had been on the market for
nine months. The chicken coop my dad had built clinched
the deal, and the young couple wanted to close quickly. We
didn't have time to pack everything from the house, barn,
and garage directly into a cargo container, so it was all just
temporarily stored at Extra Space Storage.

My parents told Jose to go ahead and make the deal on the farm. With the extra money we sent him, Jose would purchase a milk tank, milking machine, and a grinder for the cows' feed.

Before Jose hung up, he said, "Jeem, tell Velya I gonna wear the monkey socks she give me on the day you move here."

Velya

For 13 nights, I dreamed about our Bridgewater house. These weren't bad or sad dreams, but they did seem like important dreams in which I was supposed to be learning something. In all of the dreams, the house was totally empty. I wasn't actually in the house, but was somehow listening to all the noises one comes to identify with a home they've lived in for many years.

Jim had converted an old ironing board cupboard into a large shelved cabinet, and the black wrought-iron latch had a distinctive click. I supposed the muffled whooshing noise of the Atrium front door opening meant someone had come home and was where they belonged. I heard it all: the water pump in the basement kicking on, tiny footsteps coming down the stairs from the kids' rooms, and pecking noises on the dining room window where Bronco, the imprinted goose we incubated on the kitchen counter, tried to catch Mic's attention as we ate dinner. The dryer buzzed to indicate a load of clothes was done. The grandfather clock chimed in the living room—it was our last big purchase before starting a family. In the pantry, baby chicks huddled under a glowing heat lamp, making contented peeping sounds. The cat door under the bathroom sink banged open as Orville made an entrance into the house with a wounded chipmunk in his mouth. The top drawer of Jim's antique dresser slid open as he grabbed a clean pair of underwear to begin his day at dawn. The humming furnace, jangling car keys, and roll of aluminum foil tearing across the metal teeth of its cardboard box as someone covered up leftovers. The uniquely-winter scraping sound as snow shovel met stone walk. Matchbox cars crashed into wooden baseboards. High heels from the dress-up box shuffled across the blue kitchen floor tiles, which had been laid by Jim and Jose. For 13 nights, I dreamed these sounds and kind of levitated over the empty house.

Did the emptiness in the house signify I was starting over, starting anew? Perhaps the house represented me and my family. Furniture symbolically represents specific aspects of life, but my dream had no furniture, no possessions. Was I wiping everything clean in my own mind—ready for a new start?

Perhaps the dreams were telling me to listen carefully to my wise inner voice, to the wisdom of the human heart. There were no unpleasant sounds in any of the dreams. There was no crying, yelling, or harsh noise. Instead, as I hovered over the house and passed back and forth seamlessly from present to past, it was all wonderful. These weren't nightmares; they were more like a cataloging, as if I were taking inventory and filing something away.

CHAPTER TWENTY

Ehris

O ur years of planning had been a slow crawl, but once things were put into motion, the crawl became a sprint. We were making so many important decisions in such a short span of time. Everything that happened remains kind of a blur.

Our Brazilian friend, Aureliano, helped us schedule a 53-foot cargo container that would carry everything from our house, barn, and garage across the Atlantic Ocean to Rio de Janeiro. Its journey would take four weeks. Once Aureliano booked the container, we only had six days to prepare for its arrival. We frantically made sure everything we planned to take to Brazil would be ready to be loaded, since we were allowed only five hours to move everything from Extra Space Storage to the container.

Velya

Some people spend months poring over *Consumer Reports* and store circulars when they decide to buy a new washing machine. I've never been one of those people.

Four days before the container arrived, Jim called me from his final construction job and said, "You and Ehris have to get over to Lew White Appliances. I didn't realize until just now that all of our appliances need to be ordered today, or they won't be delivered in time to make it on the container."

We flew into the store at 11:00 A.M., and it was closing at noon. I informed the unfortunate salesman, "We need to pick out appliances quickly. Really quickly!"

"Okay," he said, calmly reaching for a product catalog. "What are you looking for? A fridge?"

"We don't just need a fridge. We need a whole house full of appliances for Brazil, and we need them delivered to our storage place by Tuesday morning."

"Brazil?" he questioned. "Are you Brazilian?"

"No," I responded.

"Do you have family in Brazil?"

"No," I sighed. "We just want to try something new, but this stuff has to get loaded on our cargo container on Tuesday."

"Tuesday?!" he exclaimed. "Let's get a move on!"

Now that I think about it, if this guy worked on commission, I guess he wasn't an unfortunate salesman. He basically picked out everything as Ehris and I nodded and trotted along behind him. When it was all over, he was out of breath and had to sit down. He told us that the appliances should arrive in time, and gave us the dimensions so Jim could start planning the cabinet and counter layout. When we got back in the car, I asked Ehris, "What'd ya think of the dishwasher?"

She laughed and said, "I don't think I ever really saw it."

"Yeah, neither did I. I don't even know what kind of refrigerator we got! Did we get the freezer on the bottom, like the guy recommended?"

"I have no idea," Ehris said, "I just know everything we got is white. I guess it'll be a surprise when we open the boxes!"

Next, we had to race over to Costco. Isabela had me petrified that once we left American soil, we would never again see a piece of aluminum foil or a Ziploc bag. We chucked boxes of garbage bags, dishwasher soap, Baggies, plastic wrap, and knockoff Tupperware into the cart. Jose had recommended that we get a monstrous spotlight in case of surprise cow birthings or "visits from bad guys," and luckily, Costco had one left. In Ponte Nova, there isn't anything like a Walmart where you can just walk in and grab underwear, socks, garbage cans, plastic hangers, or a toaster. To find a store like that, you would need to go to São Paulo or Rio de Janeiro, which are over eight hours away.

CHAPTER TWENTY-ONE

Ehris

On the day the cargo container arrived, the weather was predicted to be 30 degrees and sunny; but, as Mark Twain wrote, "If you don't like the weather in New England, just wait a few minutes." The forecast changed overnight to a high temperature of six degrees. Our boxes of shearling-lined L.L. Bean boots, hats, winter jackets, gloves, and scarves were buried somewhere in our Extra Space Storage unit, so my mom and I made a speedy trip to Target for some cheapo boots and jackets.

Since our house had been sold, we were staying with my mom's teacher friend, Vivian, and her husband, Jeff. I think they thought the whole Brazil move was harebrained, but they bit their tongues and offered us gloves and hats. Jeff offered to let Mic (who was home from Puerto Rico on winter break and no longer owned winter clothes) wear his fluorescent orange log-cutting pants with navy blue suspenders. I didn't know what log cutting pants were until Jeff explained, "They're indestructible. A chainsaw blade bounces off them without even leaving a mark." Mic was at least eight inches taller than Jeff, so the indestructible pants fit him like capris.

Sighing, Mic decided to wear his skinny jeans so he would be fashionable even in the six degree weather.

All of our helpers were assembled and shivering when my dad's phone rang. In frosty breaths, he explained, "That was Fernando from the container company. He said that the tractor-trailer with our container just crashed into a snowbank, and the driver's gonna be delayed."

Everyone ran to their vehicles and turned on the heat to wait. Half an hour later, the driver arrived. Aureliano pulled out a fat black marker and gave us some bad news. He said, "The container company tell me every box has to have number, and then after that is done they gonna need a list with the contents of every single box."

Aureliano told me, "Ehris, you need to type the list in English and Portuguese. You have to say how much everything cost in dollars and *reals*." We had absolutely no idea what was in our boxes or how much the stuff was worth. They had been packed in a chaotic frenzy and labeled generically, like *kitchen; doilies, or however you spell it;* and *pantry stuff*. A few were actually labeled specifically, like *keyboards and Ehris's high heels, Veal's bras,* and *Polish Stoneware butter dish lid and George Foreman grill.*

When Aureliano opened up the back of his van, it revealed the two giant boxes he was going to ship on our container. Unlike our used cardboard boxes held together with packing tape, he had constructed perfect plywood boxes with hinges and screws, and four little wheels on the bottom for easy maneuvering. They were clearly numbered and labeled. He had neglected to tell us about these plywood boxes and gaped at our storage space, overflowing with boxes of every shape and size. Some things weren't even in boxes, like the six cases of baby wipes and industrial-size box of Lactaid. We would have to assign numbers to the stone cherubs, couches, rakes, post-hole diggers, shovels, saddles, porch swings, cement benches, carjacks, and pieces of plywood, copper tubing, and foam insulation my dad had bought to build a solar-powered water heater.

We had to make sure *not* to assign numbers to all the illegal things we were bringing. Technically, it's illegal to bring gas-powered items to Brazil (the Brazilian government wants you to buy those items in Brazil). My dad sneakily parked his white construction van so it was blocking the truck driver's side mirror. He didn't want him to see the two golf carts, compressor, chainsaws, weed whacker, and generator as they emerged from the storage space and were buried in the cargo container. There were rumors that containers were sometimes x-rayed in port, but we decided to take a chance.

The Lew White Appliance delivery truck arrived just as we were about to begin loading. Two seconds later, my dad's landscaper friend, Ed, showed up with an antique hand-crank corn grinder and the type of plow you pull with a mule hanging off his pickup truck.

"What are you doing here, Ed?" my mom asked.

"Didn't Jim tell you he's bringing this stuff to Brazil?" he answered.

"Uh, no, but thanks for bringing it over."

Loading the container in six-degree weather was bad, but it was even worse because we had two stuffed storage units. One was conveniently located at ground level. To reach the other unit on the second floor, you had to take a freight elevator and get out at level three. Then you had to turn a little dial with a timer for the lights to come on and walk down to the end of the dim hallway. I hated going to this storage unit alone. Every time I walked to Unit 37, I felt like I was in a CSI episode. I imagined body parts and torture devices behind every metal sliding door.

When we signed up for the storage space, the owner had told us we were not allowed to store food, stolen items, drugs, or dead bodies. We learned that as a special perk, the manager actually got to live inside one of the storage units. Her name was Belinda, and I imagined her watching TV in her little windowless home.

Our strategy was to empty the upstairs storage unit first, then move on to the other one. Mic, a Brazilian guy named Lei (pronounced "Lay"), and I took charge of emptying the space, loading the items onto rolling carts and sending them down in the elevator. Lei looked like he was freezing, and he didn't have any gloves. I told him we had an extra pair in the car, but he said, "No, I okay." I thought he was trying to act manly, but I didn't know what was so manly about not wear-ing gloves. Mic unlocked the storage unit door, and we were assaulted by a wooden carousel horse, 27 boxes of my mom's teaching supplies, rocking chairs, a bean bag chair, pillows, blankets, spice racks, a handmade yarn doll from Scotland, my Barbies, and the toy horse stables my dad had made for Mic and me. That was just the first layer.

After loading up the rolling carts, we had the delightful task of sending them down in the elevators. You might think, *Oh, that's no problem! Just wheel it in and push the button.* But for some reason, when Extra Space Storage was built, the elevator people didn't account for the size of the rolling carts when they conferred about which size elevator to install. The freight elevator was the size of a regular human elevator. To get the rolling cart into the elevator, you had to jump in the elevator, press the "hold door open" button, jump out, wheel the cart inside, get hit by the closing doors, and then angle the cart so the doors could close. Before the doors closed, though, you would have to remember to push the "Floor 1" button. We had to do this over 20 times. Lei (whose hands were turning purple) finally accepted a pair of gloves.

Along with his two plywood boxes, Aureliano had brought a few bundles of asphalt roof shingles. Every single roof in Brazil is made out of clay tiles, and not many people know what shingles are. We loved the beautiful clay tiles, and were even going to put a tile roof on our Brazilian chicken coop. Aureliano loved the novelty of asphalt shingles, and couldn't wait to surprise his family with an asphalt-roofed gated entrance at the head of the dirt driveway that led to their *fazenda*.

The temperature was hovering at zero degrees. As the wind whipped down the storage-space alley, I stood in the rear of the container with a fat black marker and shouted the numbers and supposed contents down to my mom, which she recorded on a clipboard with mittenless hands. She and I had planned to keep our eyes peeled for some of the boxes that contained our winter clothes and pull them aside, but that idea went down the tubes, since we could barely keep up with the box brigade. This process went on for about three hours. Every 15 minutes or so, my dad would emerge from the container, looking panicked as he surveyed how much more we had to cram in. My mom and I were pretty sure that we were going to run out of room, but my dad was a little more optimistic. Mic, shivering in his skinny jeans, didn't care to hypothesize.

In the rush to empty our house, we hadn't been able to logically organize the storage space. So, when we pulled everything out of the units, it was haphazardly disorganized. We were running out of space and time. There came a point at which sacrifices had to be made.

"I feel like we're in the Donner Party," my mom said dramatically. "This is just like when they were crossing the snowy Sierra Nevadas and had to eliminate items to lighten the load on the wagon train!"

Through chattering teeth, I said, "Stop with the history lesson! At least we're not cannibals."

As the five-hour mark neared, there was more cramming and less care taken. My mom cringed as the antique red radio cabinet she had hand-finished was scratched on a metal sled (why were we bringing sleds to Brazil?) and the back panel popped off. When we were packing up our house, I had come up with the brilliant idea of putting all our plastic hangers into this empty radio cabinet. When the back panel came off, over 100 hangers exploded onto the icy pavement. Everyone took turns hurling them into the nooks and crannies of the container. We made sure that Aureliano's boxes, Isabela's mom's new washing machine, and the tools Jose had asked my dad to buy made it on board.

We took inventory of what had been forsaken: four bikes, half of Mic's bed, the marble top of a Victorian dresser, an antique loveseat my parents had salvaged from a house they had flipped, a wicker armoire, and my bean bag chair. My dad had offered a Toro self-propelled lawnmower to Isabela's father, who lived in Connecticut, and he had gratefully accepted.

We all watched as the tractor-trailer rumbled down the road. It finally seemed real. There was no turning back.

Velya

We gave ourselves 24 hours to recover, then got started on the itemized container list. Of course, we nominated Ehris to do the typing. Although Ehris's Portuguese was very good, there were a few items that even she didn't know how to translate, and she couldn't find the translations online. These were items that you wouldn't normally see in Brazil: my childhood Flexible Flyer sled, the Slovakian spice racks, baby wipes, the porch swing, Jim's drill press, snow shovels, a bucket with attached calf nipples, cow magnets, and a fishing tackle box. She emailed our Portuguese teacher, Samantha, for help. One thing that really made Portuguese difficult for Jim and me was that so many Portuguese words have multiple meanings. For instance: the word *macaco* can mean monkey, car jack, or ape. *Banco* can mean bank, bench, car seat, stool, or church pew. *Prego* means nail or to pawn. *Bomba* can mean pump or bomb. Ehris would snort, "Are you kidding? So that means that if every Portuguese word only had one meaning, you and Daddy would be fluent?"

Then came attaching a value to each of the items. Ehris typed away in front of Vivian and Jeff's cozy woodstove. Jim and Jeff were in the living room watching TV while Vivian and I gabbed away about school gossip. Every once in a while, Ehris would sing out, "How much is the blue wheelbarrow worth?" Somebody would shout back a random number and she would record it.

By the end of the six-page, single-spaced, four-column list, Ehris's singing was turning to snarling. "What about the hanging blue and green glass chandelier that hung outside on the deck over the table?"

"Uhh," Jim responded. "We had a blue and green glass chandelier? I don't remember that."

Ehris said, "Daddy, it doesn't matter if you don't remember it! Just tell me a price!"

"Mommy, how much is that stone birdbath worth?" she asked me.

I answered, "Oh, I love that stone birdbath! Remember the day I looked in the window of that antique store by the place where we had lunch that time, where they had the chicken salad with grapes in it…."

"Mommy!" Ehris cried. "Come on! Stop dorkin' around! Just give me a price!"

"How much are those dog beds from Costco worth?" Ehris asked wearily.

Vivian cheerfully exclaimed, "Oh! You have dog beds from Costco? Do you like them? We keep meaning to get one for Bubbles to put by the woodstove!"

Ehris was ready to pull a Hansel and Gretel and shove us all, except for Jeff, into the cozy woodstove. There were 179 boxes and 213 loose items. Ehris emailed the list to Aureliano.

Next on my list of tasks was arranging to ship our pets: Sylvia (a Great Dane), Chauncey (a Cairn terrier), and Harry (a cat). I knew exactly what was required for the paperwork, which I couldn't complete until we had booked our flights. Of course, we knew that all three of the animals would have to fly in kennels. Before we sold the house, I ordered and received a 700-series kennel for Sylvia. The 700-series is designed for giant breeds like Newfoundlands, mastiffs, and Great Danes. When it came, I joked, "A whole Brazilian family could live in this kennel!" Ehris tried it out to prove my point, and was amazed at how roomy it was. It was now in Vivian and Jeff's garage.

Normally, we flew TAM Airlines to Brazil, so this was who I contacted first. However, phone calls to TAM and five other airlines revealed the following distressing and illogical information: airport temperatures had to be between 40 and 75 degrees in order for animals to be able to fly in the cargo compartment of a passenger plane. Without being an Einstein, it was pretty easy to figure out that February at a New York airport would probably not be within that temperature range, but animals could fly on a cargo plane out of Kennedy Airport in February for a nominal fee of $6,000 each, one way. They would also be permitted to fly one-way out of a New York airport if we hired a pet broker for $6,000. Our round-trip flights, as three humans, were going to cost $3,000!

I also learned that even if we found a flight, Sylvia could only get as far as São Paulo. Her mandatory 700-series kennel couldn't fit on the connecting flight to Belo Horizonte. We decided that if necessary, Jim would leave a week ahead of us, pick up the Gol in Ponte Nova, and drive the 435 mile, nine hour trip to the São Paulo airport to pick us up. Of course, it would have been easier just to rent a car from São Paulo, but Ponte Nova was so remote that we couldn't find a rental car company willing to let us drop it off there, or in any town within a three-hour radius. I learned that because of Harry's small size, he would be allowed to go in a carry-on kennel under our seats; but having experienced his incessant meowing on trips to the vet, we decided it would be a better idea to put him in the cargo hold, so we wouldn't be tossed out the emergency exit door by our fellow passengers. I couldn't believe that we had gotten this far in our journey only to be thwarted by airline policy. I sat in the living room with everyone, holding my head and brainstorming ways we could affordably get the animals to Brazil. Jeff, who had a pilot's license, even suggested chartering a private plane. Discouraged, I fell asleep with container lists and dog kennels in my nightmares.

Jeff came down to breakfast and announced, "I've had a revelation." Since he was a Continental Airlines first-class frequent flier, he had access to their exclusive VIP lounge. The last time he'd been in the special lounge at Newark Airport in New Jersey, he remembered seeing a sign that read, "Need to ship a pet? Call Continental QuikPak!"

Jeff handed me the paper he had printed out. I called Continental Airlines QuikPak and spoke with Southern-accented Patrick. He was a chatty fellow, and told me, "You know, honey, other airlines are gonna try and tell ya they can help ya, but don't believe 'em. We're the only folks who can help ya out, and I've been doin' this job for 20 years."

I was immediately relieved, and gave him the vital statistics on Chauncey, Harry, and Sylvia.

Patrick asked, "Honey, are Sylvia's ears cropped?"

I remember thinking how weird that question was, and didn't know what the correct response was. I hesitated for a second before answering, "No."

Patrick responded, "Well, that's great news, honey! Those extra inches would have done you in." He explained that the extra ear height would have prevented her from fitting in the 700-series, the largest kennel made.

Good old Patrick came through. He booked Ehris, Chauncey, Sylvia, Harry, and me on a direct Continental flight to São Paulo. Jim would leave a week before and pick us up at the airport, since Sylvia couldn't fit on the connecting flight. Patrick told me where to drop the animals off once we got to Newark Airport. He advised that it would be easiest to pay in cash, and the price would be $1,500. Patrick gave me suggestions to make the process easier for the animals. He told me the 700 Series kennel was perfect for Sylvia, and to get a 300 Series for Harry, and a 400 for Chauncey, at Petco.

"Honey, now listen to me, 'cause I've been doin' this for 20 years. For your kitty, you're gonna wanna get him a small disposable litter box. They sell 'em at Petco. Just before ya leave, wear some socks around the house, and put 'em in the kennels. The socks will have your scent on them, and that'll be comfortin' to the pets. Make sure ya get enough food for each of 'em 'cause someone'll feed them durin' the flight. Write out the instructions and tape 'em to the food. Each animal needs a food and water bowl. The folks at QuikPak will give ya ice cubes to put in the water bowl. They'll melt during the flight, and your furry friends will be just fine. Get lots of newspaper, and line the bottoms of all the kennels to soak up any accidents. Whateva you do, don't use any colored newspaper. The colors will go into their little paws and they'll have a problem. Don't tranquilize 'em—the airline won't take 'em if they suspect they've been tranquilized. Drop 'em off three hours before the flight. Have a great trip, honey, and God bless ya."

Thank goodness! I was now able to schedule the animals' veterinary exams, which had to be perfectly choreographed to synchronize with the correct dates for the state veterinarian paperwork—and, ultimately, the Brazilian Consulate documents. I booked an earlier flight for Jim. He would be leaving out of Kennedy Airport a week before Ehris, the animals, and me. It stunk that we couldn't all travel together, but there was no other way to make it work.

We booked round-trip tickets because dear friends of ours were getting married in June, and we wanted to return from Brazil to be there for their Bridgewater wedding. Mic had gone back to the University of Puerto Rico, but would meet us in Connecticut in the summer, and the animals would remain in Brazil. Jim had a few Urban Crossroads jobs lined up for June, so we would stay in Connecticut for about a month before returning to Ponte Nova. We decided to leave Jim's tool-filled work van parked at a friend's house, along with the car we were keeping. Jim gave our Volvo to Dacio, Isabela's father.

The final days were spent on important but time-consuming details: paying the cell phone bill five months in advance, making sure there was enough money in the checking account to cover the monthly health insurance premium until we decided if we were going to get Brazilian health insurance, and "porting" our home phone number of 25 years to my cell phone. When things finally happened, they happened so suddenly that many people weren't even aware that we had sold our house. Jim had arranged for someone to take care of any small construction jobs that came up while we were away. We hadn't officially closed Urban Crossroads, because we didn't want to cut off all ties with the United States in case we had to come back for some reason. My mother was in poor health, and we didn't know what the future would bring.

Even though we were coming back to Connecticut in

June, we were invited to many farewell dinners. "You're so brave to move out of the country," our hosts would say. "We would never have the guts to leave everything familiar and start a new chapter." Five of my teacher friends arranged a going-away party for me at Vivian's house. We watched the sing-along version of *Mamma Mia* in their bubbling hot tub, whooping out the lyrics. It was so cold that ice formed on our hair, but the memory of that evening still warms my heart.

CHAPTER TWENTY-TWO

Ehris

The guy at Petco had never heard of a disposable litter box. After rummaging around in Vivian's junk cabinet, we found one of those green Styrofoam containers that hamburger meat comes in, and decided it would be good enough.

"I don't see how this is going to work," my mom said, shaking her head. "This Styrofoam thing takes up half of Harry's kennel. I know darn well the kitty litter will be everywhere by the time we get to Brazil."

"Yeah, I don't get it either," I agreed, but we dutifully filled the Styrofoam container with Tidy Cat clumping kitty litter. My mom and I took turns wearing three of my dad's old holey white socks around the house to get them "scented."

We scoured the Petco aisles for some kind of dog food that would be easy for the plane people to feed Chauncey, Sylvia, and Harry, and found these things called Buckaroo Burgers, with corny cowboys on horseback twirling lassos on the bag. If you used your imagination, the "burgers" kind of resembled dehydrated hamburger patties. My mom and I really couldn't figure out how this was all going to work.

I asked many times, "Wait, are the people going to be

down in the cargo part to give them food? Are they going to be just the regular flight attendants, or do they have special animal feeder people? I didn't even know there was a way to get *down* to the cargo part from the plane cabin!"

Still at Petco, we decided that Harry would need a collar and ID tag in case he escaped at the airport or in the plane. We went to the little self-service engraving machine and debated about whether to get him the Pirates of the Caribbean tag, the fluorescent pink heart shape, the blue reflective bone, or the plain old silver nametag. Well, we really didn't debate about this, because the whole time we knew we were going to get the plain old silver one. Sylvia and Chauncey already had tags, but theirs had our Bridgewater address. There wasn't enough room to get *Fazenda das Perobas, the road between Ponte Nova and Barra Longa, the 8th kilometer, Ponte Nova, Minas Gerais, Brazil, 3543200* engraved on the tiny tag, so we just put my mom's cell phone number. If they had escaped *en route*, I don't know where they would have wound up.

I collected stacks of newspaper and sorted through each and every sheet to make sure it was only black and white. Sylvia's kennel could have held three editions of the Sunday *New York Times*. My mom bagged and clearly labeled their food while I clipped the plastic food and water bowls onto the kennel doors. She put all of the authenticated documents in her special striped purple vinyl accordion folder, along with our passports, plane tickets, birth certificates, 401K paperwork, emergency phone numbers, car titles, teaching certification, and bank account information. Everybody grew to hate this accordion folder, including her, but it held vitally important information, and she was ridiculously paranoid about losing it.

The day before my mom and I left, my dad called from Brazil with our new bank account information and number. He had opened it in the town of Matipó with Aureliano's help. We wired money to the account. Then my dad called again, saying he needed us to go to Ring's End and buy five pounds of galvanized sheetrock screws, an economy pack of razor blades for his box cutter knife, and a large box of staples for his staple gun. Vivian had convinced my mom that she couldn't live without cast iron frying pans, now that we would be cooking on a gas stove rather than a ceramic cook-top electric one. We found three graduated-size ones at TJ Maxx. At Walmart, we bought two giant boxes of mothballs to scatter in the van and car to hopefully discourage mice from spending the winter in our vehicles. We stored our remaining winter clothes in Vivian and Jeff's barn, corralled Sylvia and Chauncey on the sun porch, threw a comforting scented sock into each kennel, sprinkled the mothballs all over the inside of the car, and waited for the *I'll Drive* guy to bring us to Newark Airport.

CHAPTER TWENTY-THREE

Velya

We were instructed to drop the animals off at Newark Airport's QuikPak three hours before our flight to São Paulo. So, my neurotic former self arranged for *I'll Drive* to get us to the airport six and a half hours before our departure. When the passenger van arrived, Justin, who had driven us many times before, popped out of the driver door with sunglasses on top of his head. He always reminded me of a conceited and cocky Robert Downey, Jr., but he was the ideal guy for this situation because he was easy-going and chatty.

"Hey, how ya doin', man?" Justin nodded to Jeff as they dragged Sylvia's Shetland-pony sized kennel out of the garage. As I rolled our suitcases over to the van, I overheard him exclaim, "Yo, bro, what the hell is going in this thing?"

He got his answer when Ehris came through the sun porch door with our 140-pound Great Dane on a hot pink leash.

"Dude, that's quite a dog you got there!" Justin said admiringly as Ehris led her down the stone path. I prepared to put Sylvia in the kennel, but he waved me away and said, "Nah, she doesn't have to go in there. She can just be loose in the van."

"Are you serious?" I asked in surprise as Justin casually preened his shoulder-length rocker hair.

"She can sit on the back seat," he replied. Stroking Sylvia's massive black and white head he declared, "Hey, big girl, you don't wanna be cooped up. You wanna be free!"

Jeff hugged us goodbye and advised Justin to stop at a certain rest stop near the airport to let the dogs walk around and go to the bathroom one last time. Harry sulked in his cat carrier on top of the suitcases. Chauncey alternated between my lap and Ehris's lap, and Sylvia took up the entire third row. As Justin closed the doors to the van, it was as if the doors were closing on a chapter of our lives.

Ehris

As expected, my mom and Justin never stopped yakking. Justin asked us to bring him back a bottle of *cachaça* in June. He offered us pieces of pink Dubble Bubble gum as he chomped away and constantly flipped through radio stations in search of the latest traffic report. My mom asked, "Justin, how's your baby?"

Justin paused for a moment and said, "She's doing well. She's got me wrapped around her finger."

"Yeah, baby girls definitely do that," my mom agreed.

The animals were extremely quiet and well behaved—even Harry in his little plastic prison. Justin commented, "Wow, I would never know there was a Great Dane in here!"

Justin sped down the New Jersey Turnpike, weaving in and out of 12 lanes of traffic. It didn't seem like he was going to take Jeff's advice, so I asked, "Do you think we can stop someplace and let the dogs out?" He told me that there was a spot coming up in a few miles. We arrived at the rest stop, which wasn't really a rest stop at all. It was getting dark, which made this place look even creepier. It was kind of a circular driveway in the middle of the city, with a patch of dirty, garbage-strewn grass.

"This looks like somewhere the Mafia would dump dead bodies," my mom muttered. She and I got out of the van. I held Sylvia's leash while she held Chauncey's, and we walked down the strip of dying grass. There were about seven parked cars at this "rest stop," and as we walked by, the eyes of the people inside the vehicles followed us—until they glimpsed intimidating Sylvia.

I walked back to the van first, and thought I was seeing things. Where Sylvia had been sitting, there was a big pile of stuff, and I wasn't really sure what it was. I quietly gasped. As my mom neared the van, I whispered, "What's on the seat!?"

"What?" she asked loudly, squinting at me. "What are you talking about?"

"The seat!" I pointed. "Look at it! I think someone threw up!"

"Shh!" my mom hissed. "Let me see!"

Sure enough, it was a pile of vomit bigger than Chauncey. Much bigger than Chauncey.

Velya

Justin called from the driver's seat, "Did you say someone threw up?"

"No, no, everything's fine," I reassured him.

He looked satisfied with this answer, put the van in drive, and went back to chomping on his gum and changing the radio stations.

I whispered, "Ehris! What are we going to do?"

Ehris whispered back, "I don't know! What do you think?"

I casually glanced over the back of my seat and almost fainted. There was a mound of very chunky barf that was made up of chicken legs, carrots, and other unidentifiable stuff. It was about the size and shape of a baby seal. Amazingly, it didn't smell. When Sylvia threw up, she must have done it silently.

"We can't tell him!" I admonished in a whisper.

Honest Ehris whimpered, "We have to tell him! How are we going to hide a mountain of vomit?"

"I don't know. But if we tell him, he'll never let us out of this van, and we'll never make the flight!" I reasoned in a frenzied whisper. "Daddy will be driving around Brazil looking for us for the rest of his life! We'll be stranded at Newark with two dogs, a cat, and 50 pounds of screws and razor blades. We only have three Buckaroo Burgers, Ehris! Justin won't notice the barf." Looking back on it, I have no idea why we didn't just confess. It was totally out of character for us to do something like this, but it just felt like we couldn't let anything stop us from getting to Brazil. At the time, Ehris and I truly thought that we would escape that van with Justin none the wiser. We would be on the plane by the time he got back to I'll Drive headquarters and discovered the puke.

We then came up with an elaborate whispered plan. Ehris would hop out of the van first as I held Chauncey and Sylvia's leashes. She would grab the purple suitcase that was in the front seat, while I would gently shove Sylvia and Chauncey out the van door. Ehris would then shut the door with lightning speed, so fast that Justin wouldn't even know what was happening. As Ehris, Chauncey, Sylvia, and Harry ran to the QuikPak drop-off, I would keep Justin talking and distracted as we removed the bags from the rear of the van.

Too soon, we arrived at the airport and had to put the foolproof plan into action.

Ehris

As planned, I hopped out of the van while it was still moving, grabbed the rolling purple suitcase, and caught the dogs' leashes as my mom frantically threw them at me. She jumped out and I slammed the van door, confident that the vomit would not be spotted. Somehow, with superhuman powers, I managed to hold both Sylvia and Chauncey, my backpack, and Harry's plastic carrier. We rushed to the QuikPak entrance, leaving the purple suitcase on the sidewalk for my mom to deal with.

I entered QuikPak and put Harry and the backpack on the linoleum floor. I told the woman at the desk that I was here to drop off my pets for a flight to Brazil. After I explained why we were moving to Brazil, and that no, we weren't Brazilian, she proceeded to look up our reservation on the computer. Since we wanted to have a stress-free airport experience, we had allowed ourselves extra time at

Newark for a nice dinner and time to change money, make our farewell phone calls, and stroll through duty-free. We had it all planned out that once we got on the plane and got settled in our reserved bulkhead seats, we were going to share my iPod headphones, and, at just the right moment, play Andrea Bocelli and Sara Brightman's poignant duet, "Time to Say Goodbye," as we said goodbye to our Connecticut lives.

The woman found our information on the computer and asked one of her co-workers to make sure the kennels, which Justin had lugged in, were securely assembled. The co-worker, a short blond man named Floyd, was very helpful. He checked the sizes of the kennels and recorded them on a little notepad. Floyd looked at Harry's kennel and asked, "Did someone have a little accident?" I followed his gaze and saw that Sylvia's vomit had shot all over the kennel.

It was clearly visible, but still in lying-to-Justin mode, I answered sweetly, "No, I don't think so!"

He went back to the computer to verify that the kennel sizes were correct. After a minute, he said, "Oh, you have a problem."

"What?" I asked distractedly, spotting vomit on Sylvia's leash.

"You have the wrong size for your Great Dane. It's too small for her."

I told him calmly, "No, that can't be. My mom talked to Patrick at Continental and he told her that was the size to buy. He said that since Sylvia's ears aren't cropped, it would be fine. The 700 series kennel is the largest there is."

Floyd shook his head sadly. "I'm sorry, miss, but you're going to need some kennel extenders."

"Kennel extenders? What?" I asked him. By now, my mom had been outside for a while, and I knew that once she came into QuikPak she was going to freak out about the kennel problem.

He then entered some more information on the computer and disclosed, "Oh, no! You have the wrong size for your cat and little dog, too."

"What?" I exclaimed. "Are you kidding?" I was beginning to think that Patrick was a big liar.

Velya

Meanwhile, back on the sidewalk, I was having problems of my own. Big problems. I went over to get a rolling metal luggage cart from the self-service machine, where they were all lined up against the side of the building. At every other airport in the world, these carts are free for the using. However, you have to pay for them in the United States. Not wanting to bring American change to Brazil, the smallest thing I had was a $20 bill. I asked Justin if he had change for a 20, but the only thing he had was a dollar bill. I traded him the 20 for the dollar and told him to keep the change. I returned with the luggage cart just as Justin reached into the back of the van to grab the suitcases. He recoiled his arm in shock and yelped, "What's this? What's on my fingers?" I knew the jig was up.

Sylvia's throw-up hadn't confined itself to the third row. It had shot over the back of the seat and splattered all over the suitcases. Justin opened the side door and cried, "Whoa! What happened back here?" Now, with the streetlights shining on the pile, it looked even bigger and chunkier. Justin asked, "Well, what are we going to do about this?"

I acted totally shocked, like it was the first time I had seen this mess. "Oh! Do you have any paper towels?" *Like a whole case of them?*

"No, I don't. But I do have a used paper plate," he said through gritted teeth. We both knew what that meant. With my bare hands, I started scooping up the barf, putting it on the paper plate, and walking to the sidewalk garbage can. It took about nine trips before the seat was a little less disgusting. We parted as amicably as possible, but didn't shake hands. I wheeled the heavy luggage cart down the sidewalk with my elbows, keeping my vomity hands raised, comforted to know that Ehris had everything under control with QuikPak.

Ehris

My mom finally came through the automatic sliding doors pushing a luggage cart with her hands up in the air. I could tell by her face that Justin had discovered the problem. I feigned cheerfulness while glancing at her hands, and burst out, "Sylvia's kennel is too small. So is Chauncey's. And Harry's. Where were you?"

Her expression changed to horror as she exclaimed, "What? Patrick said they were the right size! I just cleaned up all that vomit with my bare hands!"

I cringed and looked to Floyd to tell my mom what was going on. However, he had disappeared into the back room.

He came back with a handful of sanitary wipes, intended for Harry's kennel. Once he got a look at my mom's hands, he gave her one, and then another, and another. He kindly wiped off Harry's kennel while Larry, a guy behind the counter, gave her a thorough explanation.

"So, ma'am, here's what's happening. Your Great Dane needs three more inches of headroom in her kennel."

My mom screeched, "You've got to be kidding me! She could jump down, turn around, and pick a bale of cotton in there." She wasn't exaggerating. This thing was bigger than a washing machine, and Sylvia had plenty of space to stand up. She could have had friends over. She could have had a party in there.

"Ma'am, this isn't my rule, but Continental requires all animals to have three inches of headroom," Larry explained. "There's a possibility that we may be able to help you out. In our back room, I think we used to have a set of kennel extenders."

"And if you don't *have* these kennel extenders?" my mom asked.

He said, "Then we would have to order a set from Seattle."

"How long would *that* take?" she questioned.

"From Seattle to Newark...about two weeks," Larry told us.

My mom and I gasped and shuddered.

"Ma'am, let me go take a look in the back room for those extenders."

My mom declared, "I'll tell you what, Larry. If you don't come back with the extenders, then you better come back with a doctor, because I'm going to have a heart attack right here on your QuikPak floor. My husband is going to be waiting for us in Brazil tomorrow morning, I have no way to get a hold of him, our animals' paperwork from the consulate is valid only for today, and I followed all of Patrick's instructions to a T."

CHAPTER TWENTY-FOUR

Ehris

As departing planes rumbled the night sky, I stared at the cheesy kitten calendar hanging behind the QuikPak counter. I couldn't believe that the headroom in Sylvia's kennel was delaying our flight check-in, as well as our dreams.

Larry returned from the back room, holding what looked like two-by-fours.

"*Those* are the kennel extenders?" my mom questioned. She muttered to me, "Oh, my god! Daddy could have screwed this stupid wood onto the kennel in ten minutes."

Floyd said, "You're going to have to take a drive to Petco to get larger kennels for the little dog and the cat."

Harry hadn't made a peep in about three hours. I looked in his carrier to make sure he was still alive. Underneath the newspaper, tipped-over Styrofoam meat tray, and two cups of scattered kitty litter, I could see him breathing.

My mom said to Floyd, "I don't have a car. We were dropped off here, so how am I going to get to Petco? What about if we move the cat to the little dog's kennel? Then we would just need a kennel for the little dog, right?"

Floyd cried, "Oh! You might be in luck. I think I remember seeing a 500-series kennel that someone left in the back room. Let me go take a look."

Slowly emphasizing every word, my mom said, "I can't believe this is happening, Ehris. What are we going to do?"

"I guess if we have to, we can ask Jeff to come and pick us up," I suggested.

"Yeah, but Daddy already left Jose's house, and is on his way to the airport." My dad didn't have a cell phone yet, because we hadn't had time to figure out which provider would offer service in our remote section of Ponte Nova.

"I guess we can't just cross out the date and pencil in a new one on the Brazilian Consulate documents," I said sarcastically.

Hours went by—literally. While Chauncey made friends with every single person who came in and Sylvia became the QuikPak celebrity, I peeked through a postcard-sized window in a metal door to check on the progress (or lack of progress) on the extenders. Six men with one battery drill were huddled over Sylvia's kennel. I tried to make eye contact to see if I could at least get a thumbs-up or thumbs-down, so we would know if we had any chance of going to Brazil that night. All six guys looked up at me and shrugged their shoulders.

It was getting close to check-in time for our flight. A very nice woman behind the counter told us that she would call the Continental check-in desk and let them know we were here, but delayed in QuikPak. I looked through the tiny window to the back room and saw that the entire kennel was now dismantled. Floyd came out and said that they could put the extenders on, but didn't know if the door would close.

"Can't we just like hold it closed with a bungee cord?" I asked hopefully, but he shook his head and said no.

We waited and waited, still unsure of what was to come. No one had given us an update for a while. Finally, Floyd emerged from the back room and said that he had found a 500-series kennel for Chauncey. We had been at QuikPak for six hours when the woman behind the counter got a crackly static signal on her walkie-talkie and Larry's voice boomed, "It's a go. The Great Dane is going to Brazil. Over." As relieved as we were, Larry was about six feet away, and could have easily come out and told her (and us) the news.

Floyd and one of his colleagues got to work. They told us that they would need to remove the newspaper and replace it with Wee-Wee Pads.

I yelped, "But Patrick said to put in newspaper!"

As they removed the newspaper and the tipped-over kitty litter container in Harry's kennel, my mom explained, "Patrick said to put a kitty litter pan in the cat's kennel." She handed them the carefully labeled bags of Buckaroo Burgers, and they handed them right back. "Let me guess, Patrick was wrong on that one, too?" she asked, irritated.

Out came the food bowl and my dad's holey socks. Patrick had lied about everything. It came time to take Harry out of his kennel and switch him into Chauncey's original 400-series. I had dreaded this moment, because I expected that Harry was going to scratch their eyes out and escape through the automatic sliding doors. Instead, he meekly allowed them to pick him up and gently place him in his temporary home. Floyd plastered "This End Up" and "Live Animals On Board" labels, complete with all of their iden-tification information, on all three kennels. The only thing

Patrick had been correct about was the ice cubes, which Floyd plopped into their water bowls. The entire experience had been extremely frustrating, but the QuikPak employees were very gentle and comforting with the animals. At the counter, my mom discovered the last of Patrick's lies. As she attempted to pay with the cash that Patrick had instructed was necessary, they said that it would be much faster to just pay with a credit card. She exhaled, "Patrick said to pay with cash! He said you wouldn't accept credit cards."

The woman behind the counter finally asked, "Who *is* this Patrick?"

My mom, who though Patrick had an office somewhere at Newark Airport, said, "Patrick, your QuikPak guy who I talked to on the phone. He had a Southern accent."

"I've never heard of him. He's probably based out of Atlanta," the woman answered. "Now I understand your frustration!"

It was now after 10:00 P.M., and Floyd escorted us up to the Continental check-in desk. He wished us a nice flight and assured us that they would take good care of the pets.

CHAPTER TWENTY-FIVE

Ehris

Floyd left as we began the check-in process. We took our suitcases off of the luggage cart, and I handed our passports and e-Tickets to the check-in woman. As I took a closer look at the suitcases, I noticed that Sylvia's vomit had gotten over all of them, too. My mom asked for paper towels as the woman looked the e-Tickets over and responded sternly, without glancing up, "No, we don't have paper towels, and the gate is already closed for this flight."

"What? The gate's *closed*?" we said simultaneously.

"Can you open it?" I asked.

She said firmly, "No. You're supposed to check in at least an hour and half before the flight."

My mom informed her, "Listen, we've been in Continental QuikPak for the last six hours trying to drop our animals off. They called you to let you know we were here."

"It doesn't matter. The gate's closed. We can't open it."

My mom said, "Look, we're flying to Brazil tonight with three pets who are now being loaded on the plane. I think you better let us talk to your supervisor."

The woman jogged stiffly over to the supervisor's door and knocked three times. A lady in a red suit came out, and there were a lot of animated hand gestures and nodding in our direction. Red Suit clicked over in her authoritative high heels, got our version of the story, and called the gate.

"They're holding the plane for you. Take your bags and get over there right now!" she commanded.

I asked, "You mean take our suitcases with us? Like through security?"

She rooted, "Yes, go now! I hope you make it!"

My mom grabbed her purse, quilted carry-on, and two suitcases. I grabbed the other two suitcases, my backpack, and the laptop. We ran towards security. Well, not really. We trotted as fast as humanly possible while carrying this much stuff. In order to reach security, we had to go downstairs—either down actual stairs or down an escalator. I decided that the escalator would be faster, so I threw both suitcases in front of me and held the backpack and laptop. My mom's flowered suitcase somehow got caught on the side of the escalator. That was it. I'd had enough. I soccer-kicked the suitcase as hard as I could. It was so heavy that it didn't really fly through the air—it just tumbled to the bottom. I got off the escalator with my rolling cheetah suitcase and picked up the flowered one.

My mom was already at security, taking off her flip-flops. I saw the looming baggage x-ray screen and frantically thought, *the staples! The screws! The cast iron frying pans! The razor blades! How are we going to get through security?* My thoughts went back to the flowered suitcase, which wasn't moving. I quickly examined it and discovered that my kick had totally mangled its wheels. I realized they were so twisted, I would have to carry this 150-pound suitcase the rest of the way. I heaved the cheetah and mutilated flowered suitcases onto the conveyor belt, and questioned TSA standards as they let our extremely contraband items through without a second glance.

My mom looked at her e-Ticket and howled, "Ehris, we have to make it to gate 1A!"

Gate 1A was at the very end of the concourse, of course. I grunted as I lifted up the vomity flowered suitcase with one hand, rolling the giant cheetah bag with the other down the endless hallway. My mom was lagging behind, but I couldn't stop. I couldn't look back. I couldn't talk. I could barely breathe. I concentrated on reaching the end of the hallway, and tried to ignore the shooting pains throughout my body. The cast iron frying pans banged into my ankles, and I wondered why my mom had bought these stupid things.

Finally, Gate 1A was in sight. I sighed in relief, but I shouldn't have. They were just starting to make the boarding announcements as I limped to the counter. I cheerfully greeted Gladys, the Continental check-in person at the gate. She had straightened, slicked-back hair and long red cat claws. Gladys asked snottily, "Where are your boarding passes?"

My mom explained our QuikPak predicament, and said that the supervisor had told us to go directly to the boarding gate. Gladys repeated, "Where are your boarding passes?"

"We don't have boarding passes," I told her. "Your supervisor sent us here."

She sneered, "You have to check in an hour and a half before the flight. I can't let you on the plane without boarding passes."

"An hour and a half? We're been at this airport for over six hours!" my mom exclaimed.

"You should have come and checked in. I can't let you on the plane."

My mom had stayed pretty calm up until this point. "Number one," she listed as she held up one index finger, "the QuikPak woman called the check-in desk and let them know that we were here and what was going on. Number two," she said, dramatically raising an additional finger, "we didn't know until 20 minutes ago that our pets were even going to be allowed on the flight. So why would we check in if we didn't know that we were actually going to make the plane?"

Gladys smirked, "I know all about the situation, and I told the supervisor no. So why are you here?"

Through clenched teeth, my mom said, "The supervisor told us to come directly to the gate!"

Gladys dismissed us as if we were annoying gnats. "Go sit down and *maybe*, after I'm done checking in the other people who arrived on time, *maybe* I'll find you a seat. But don't count on it."

We shot daggers out of our eyes at Gladys and collapsed onto the plastic seats. I was pretty sure Gladys was full of it, because we knew our animals were on the plane. What was Continental Airlines going to do with an unaccompanied Great Dane, Cairn terrier, and cat once the plane landed in São Paulo? I also knew that we were caught in the middle of a power struggle between Gladys and Red Suit.

Gladys finished checking in the other people, filed her nails, and re-applied her blood-red lipstick. She had no choice but to call us over to the desk. "There's probably two seats on there," she said, gesturing to the plane with her acrylic nails. She added gleefully, "but you're not going to be anywhere near each other. Grab any seats you can find," she ordered. "Take your suitcases to the plane."

"Take the suitcases to the plane? Like the plane door?" I asked.

Gladys rolled her eyes.

I kicked the flowered suitcase down the covered ramp, trying not to kick the vomit-covered patch. We reached the plane door and were greeted by a perky flight attendant. He told us to leave our suitcases there, and they would get them into the cargo area. We got on the plane and walked past our already-occupied bulkhead seats. We found two seats next to each other in the middle section and got settled. After stowing our bags in the overhead bins and under the seats (well, not really stowing, more like shoving, cramming, and smashing), we sat down. I looked for my passport in my backpack and the laptop case, but couldn't find it. Alarmed, I asked, "Mommy, do you have my passport?"

She said, "No, you had it in your hand."

I was about to get up and head back to see if Gladys had taken it and ripped it up, but my mom spotted it between the seats, wedged under the seatbelt buckle. I looked down at the laptop case and saw something on the handle. I groaned, "Oh no, is that what I think it is?"

"Oh no, it's on my capris!" my mom yelped. "Oh no, it's on your pants!"

"Oh no, it's on my backpack!"

"Oh no, it's on my flip flops!" We both ran to the tiny bathrooms and attempted to clean ourselves up a little with paper towels and airplane soap, but it didn't really work. We went back to our seats as they made the announcement to turn off all electronic devices. We couldn't make our farewell phone calls. Andrea Bocelli was not going to serenade us as we were lifted into the cold night sky.

"What in the world is Justin going to tell I'll Drive?" my mom laughed. "I can't believe we thought he wasn't going to notice! What were we thinking? I'll Drive is probably going to blackball us."

"If they ever see our name on their caller ID, they'll never pick up," I predicted.

"What we did was pretty bad, but Justin *was* the one who said to let Sylvia loose in the van!"

"That fight between Red Suit and Gladys was pretty intense!" I grinned.

"Forget about that! How about the fact that we got through security with razor blades and five pounds of screws?"

"Do you think the animals are really on the plane?" I asked.

My mom politely asked the flight attendant if he could check that our pets were on board, and where we could pick them up once we landed. When he returned with our meals, he confirmed that they were indeed in the cargo area. There would be a Continental representative in the Guarulhos Airport who would help us.

"Well, there was one good thing about this night," I smiled.

"Oh, yeah?" my mom asked skeptically. "What was that?"

"We didn't have to pay the overage baggage fee," I snickered.

"Yeah—ha, ha, Gladys!"

Even though things had been pretty terrible, I was proud that we had remained polite and cheerful. I don't think many people would have conducted themselves as well. I didn't know if my ears were playing tricks on me, but I thought I heard faint meowing coming from below. I looked at the small monitor on the back of the seat that plotted the plane's course, and realized that we would see my dad in nine and a half hours. I closed my eyes and daydreamed about riding horses through the Brazilian wilderness.

CHAPTER TWENTY-SIX

Velya

✿

Everyone had questioned Jim's sanity and warned him about the dangers of driving across Brazil, but I had no doubt that he would be waiting for us at the airport in São Paulo. It never crossed my mind that he wouldn't be there. Jim had asked lots of Brazilians for advice on plotting the route, but no one could help. No one he met had ever driven that far, because they were too afraid of making the journey.

Ehris and I made it through passport control, customs, and baggage claim without incident. As we walked into the passenger arrival terminal, there was Jim, wearing a yellow striped polo shirt and khaki shorts, holding a cardboard sign that read "Urban," like the placards limo drivers display. It seemed perfectly normal to see him waiting for us in the Brazilian airport. It didn't feel like a momentous event that we were finally in Brazil, about to drive to our new home. We gave him a five-minute summary of our mishaps, but I don't think he really understood how close we had come to not making the flight. I think in the same way that we never doubted him being at the airport, he never doubted that we would be on the plane.

The Continental representative in the lobby directed us to the *Ministro da Agricultura* to pick up our pets. Once we finally found the building, we knew we were in the right place, because it was like trying to enter the Pentagon. While Jim parked the car, Ehris and I went into the lobby. Don't get the wrong idea of *lobby*—there weren't potted plants, cups of complimentary Keurig coffee, comfy armchairs, or magazines on coffee tables. This was more like a calm mob of men waving papers at the guard behind a horseshoe-shaped desk, trying to get permission to go somewhere. We were the only women.

It was finally our turn at the horseshoe-shaped desk. Ehris asked in Portuguese, "We're looking for our pets. Do you know where they are?"

The guard looked at her as if she had asked him an AP calculus question. "Your *pets*?"

"Yes, we just arrived on a Continental flight from Newark Airport, and our two dogs and cat were on the plane with us. We don't know where to get them," she explained.

In Portuguese, he responded in disbelief, "You brought your pets to Brazil with you? Why? Are you Brazilian? Is your father Brazilian? Do you have family in Brazil?"

Brazil's attitude about pets is totally different from America's. Dogs basically fend for themselves, and aren't allowed inside houses. Many eat out of garbage piles. As disgusting as this sounds, we once saw a dog eating the contents of a poopy diaper that had been dumped on the side of the road. Cats are barely acknowledged. We would eventually become accustomed to all the stray street dogs, but we never got over the sadness, neglect, and disregard for neutering. On one dirt road, we saw a poor dog that had a stomach tumor so big, it dragged on the ground. All over the place, there were female dogs with swollen nipples who were obviously nursing a hidden litter of puppies. Some Americans go overboard by carrying their little dogs in purses, speaking baby talk to them or dressing them up in cutesy outfits, but Brazil is at the other extreme. This guy's response was typically Brazilian.

We wheeled the three kennels into the parking lot. Sylvia attracted even more attention here than in Newark. The Gol was so small that we knew we would have to leave Chauncey and Sylvia's kennels at the airport, which didn't matter, because the dogs wouldn't be leaving Brazil, anyway. Harry stayed in his carrier, because we couldn't have a loose, jetlagged cat in the car. Amazingly, none of the animals had peed or pooped in their crates. Sylvia and Chauncey settled on the back seat with me on an old patchwork blanket from Goodwill, and Ehris sat in the passenger seat with Harry's crate on her lap.

So, in our two-door gray VW Gol filled with four suitcases, two backpacks, a laptop, a knock-off Vera Bradley purse, a Great Dane, a Cairn terrier, a deflated air mattress, a cat in a carrier, and three humans, we began the long journey to our *fazenda*.

"What's the air mattress for?" I asked Jim.

"Even though the container's not here yet, I thought it'd be fun to stay at our farm and live like pioneers for a few days until it gets here," Jim answered. "Jose wants us to come to their house first, and then he'll drive us over to see our farm. I didn't go there yet, because I wanted all of us to see it together."

"How'd you pull off the drive to the airport?" I questioned, wiping sweat off my forehead.

"I got so sick of people telling me how impossible the drive was going to be that I bought a map and plotted my own course."

"How long did it take?" Ehris asked.

"14 hours. I had to navigate around potholes the size of cars, roads that just ended, and mudslides. I had to read tiny road signs in Portuguese, and understand directions from people who had never been where I was going!"

"How'd ya find the airport?" I asked.

"I remembered a trick I learned when I was trying to find O'Hare Airport, so I did the same thing here," he explained. The last 20 miles of the trip, Jim had scanned the sky for jets, followed them, and hoped they were headed for the Guarulhos Airport. When he finally got to the airport the night before our flight arrived, he had parked the car and taken the airport shuttle to a hotel in fear that if he drove the car, he'd get lost. He woke up early to eat some *pão de queijo* and craft his little "Urban" sign.

Because of the animals, it would have been impossible for us to stop at a motel—oops, I mean hotel, because motels are just for sex in Brazil—so we had to reach Jose's house before we could sleep. We stopped about three times along our journey, and at one gas station, Sylvia drew a crowd. Great Danes are a large breed in the United States, but in Brazil, they're a non-existent breed. People tend to have smaller dogs because it's less expensive to feed them. All of the gas station men flocked to Sylvia, and were asking Jim questions in Portuguese about her. All he could say was, "Yessie, yessie, *grande cachorro*, big dog!"

Throughout the trip, Ehris and I alternated between the front and back seat of the car. Whoever sat in front got the worse part of the deal. Granted, sharing the back seat with stretched-out Sylvia was a little squishy, but it wasn't a barrel of laughs in the front seat. The occupant of the passenger seat had to hold Harry's kennel on her lap. The primary task was to keep the plastic 400-series kennel from bumping into the gear shifter as Jim sped along. Harry wasn't too responsive to our sweetly high-pitched words of encouragement. "How you doin' in there, Harry? We're almost home! Wait till you catch your first Brazilian mouse! Hang in there, buddy!" He was beginning to look a little traumatized, as were we.

It took us eight hours to reach Belo Horizonte, or as Brazilians say, "BH." This always sounded very "LA" to me, and I could never bring myself to use just the initials. We knew that the last leg of the trip, from Belo Horizonte to Ponte Nova, took three hours, so we were pretty happy with our progress. That happiness dissolved quickly as we circled the brightly-lit city for two and a half hours, lulling Ehris into a deep sleep.

For one thing, it was Carnaval, and there were roadblocks and detours everywhere. For another, Brazilian roads are not clearly marked, and the laptop-sized signs are in Portuguese. Finally, we saw a group of flashing police cars, and pulled over to attempt to ask for directions. You can imagine sleeping Ehris's surprise when Jim said urgently, "Ehris, Ehris, wake up! We need your help!" She opened her eyes to a stern-looking Brazilian cop shining a flashlight in the car window as Sylvia lunged and barked. He pointed us in the right direction, and on we traveled.

Many hours later, we wound up in Alvinópolis. After chuckling about that name for a while, we realized we were still lost. We had two choices: a paved road or a dirt road.

For some dopey reason, we took the dirt road. "Is that the sun coming up?" I asked Jim as he got out of the car to take a break. It was, indeed, the sun coming up. We had driven all night.

CHAPTER TWENTY-SEVEN

Ehris

Jose took some legal papers out of a briefcase and said, "Now we go see your fifty *hectares*." He and my dad sat at his kitchen table, looking over the documents.

My dad asked, "Jose, how many *hectares* did you just say we owned?"

"Fifty," he answered.

"Fifty? Didn't you tell me on the phone it was fifteen?" my dad asked.

"No, Jeem, I say to you, I find you a farm with fifty *hectares*," Jose responded.

With Jose's accent and the overseas phone static, my dad had misunderstood. He looked at my mom and me, and said, "Do you guys realize fifty *hectares* is equivalent to about 175 acres?"

"What? Holy mackerel! That's more than three times what we thought we had!" my mom cried.

The drive to our farm seemed endless as we crossed over to the other part of town and turned onto a dusty dirt road. We passed papaya trees, mule carts, and magenta orchids. Jose pointed and asked, "You see that fence on hill? That's where your land start."

It's hard to explain how much land 175 acres really is, but we kept saying, "You mean we own that? That, too? We own that tree over there?" This went on for about half a mile.

Velya

Nestled in the lush green mountains was a small stucco house with the ubiquitous clay tile roof. There were tropical gardens, two large ponds, and hundreds of mango trees filled with sapphire-blue parrots. Bamboo and palm trees lined the dirt driveway, and huge banana trees shaded the wraparound porch which had a ceramic tile floor and hammock hooks.

Jose pointed out the best place for Jim to build the milking *corral*. We all hiked up a steep mountain trail, and I was convinced I was getting altitude sickness. Hibiscus, cyclamen, and begonias grew wild, astonishingly bright and vibrant. Howler monkeys called from the distant tree line, and hundreds of iridescent butterflies flaunted velvet wings of electric lime and metallic blue. When we reached a plateau, I looked back over my shoulder.

"I can't believe we're finally here. Everyone was convinced we couldn't pull this off," I said, starting to tear up out of joy. I hugged Jose, who was also teary-eyed. I whispered a muffled "thank you" into his neck and felt his whiskers on my cheek.

CHAPTER TWENTY-EIGHT

Ehris

The first morning at our farm, a smiling older guy wearing an orange polo shirt appeared at the driveway gate. In Connecticut, people call before they come over, but in Brazil, people just pop in for a visit. In Portuguese, the man said his name was Guilherme, and Jose had bought our farm from him. My dad's Portuguese still hadn't improved. He extended his hand to Guilherme in greeting and said, "*Seu nomme é Jim*" (Your name is Jim). Guilherme welcomed us to the farm in a booming, bouncy voice, and repeated everything twice because he didn't think I understood what he was saying. Before he left, he shook my dad's hand and instructed, "*Se precisarem de alguma coisa, estou a suas ordens*" (If you need anything, I'm at your orders).

We ran into Guilherme almost every day in town. He always seemed happy to see us as he clapped my dad on the back and warmly hugged my mom and me. When he invited us to his apartment for lunch, we met his effervescent wife, Zoe. Even with the language barrier, we all had an instant connection.

Velya

Jose invited us to spend Carnaval at his parents' house in the mountains of Abre Campo. That day made me realize that our lives could be a pretty entertaining reality TV show. Picture a room full of Brazilian siblings and their spouses, children, grandchildren, parents, uncles, aunts, cousins, neighbors, and three bewildered Americans gathered together to celebrate the beginning of Lent.

We drove one and a half hours from Ponte Nova (New Bridge) to Abre Campo (Open Field). When we arrived at Jose's parents' house, his family cordially mobbed us. I never really knew how to greet a Brazilian. Some of them kissed you on one cheek, some kissed you on two cheeks, some just gave you a hug, and some gave you a hug and a kiss, while others simultaneously shook your hand, hugged you, and gave you two kisses and a pat on the shoulder. We learned that if you're looking for a spouse, you do the two-cheek-kiss and then go back for a third. Ehris and Mic thought it was pretty funny to imitate me as I prepared for the greetings. I sort of looked like a boxer, bobbing and weaving in the ring, not knowing what to do.

As in homes all over the world on holiday mornings, the traditional food preparation was taking place. On Brazilian *fazendas*, most women—and it does always seem to be the women—cook on a rectangular granite or tile woodstove called a *fogão a lenha*. There is no temperature dial; they adjust the heat by shoving logs into the open end of the stove. Very often, these logs are covered with ants frantically scrambling to avoid death by fire. No one uses a cookbook, timer, or measuring cups.

One *filha* (daughter) was cutting olives, one was grinding coffee beans by hand in a blue metal grinder attached to the outside of the house, and one was preparing the beans to make bean paste. Jose's mother alternately beamed with pride at her family and poured the heavily-sugared coffee, which was always offered upon entering a Brazilian home. There were no Keurigs in rural Brazil. They brewed every pot by pouring boiling water through a flannel sieve filled with ground coffee. It was then poured into a thermos. You won't find packets of stevia or Splenda, at least not in the country. They have liquid in clear plastic bottles called *Zero-Cal Adocante Dietico*.

On Brazilian farms, they use cheesecloth to strain the fresh milk before boiling, but it still doesn't have a consistent texture. One day, we went to a neighbor's house for a visit, and of course they offered us coffee. I accepted, and asked if they had any milk. The wife grabbed a small pitcher from the fridge and placed it on the table, and told me the milk had been taken from the cow just that morning. I poured some into my coffee, and immediately regretted it. There were chunks bobbing on the surface like buoys in the Atlantic! I bravely took the cup to my lips and kept my teeth together in an attempt to strain the contents. It didn't work. The gelatinous lima-bean-sized chunks of milk snuck past my teeth, and I tried not to chew them. Somehow, I choked down the entire cup of coffee, and politely declined a second.

You won't find an American-style coffee mug, either. Brazilians use *xícaras*, which are like old-fashioned American teacups with tiny handles. The drinking glasses are very small, and if you find larger ones, they're called *copo Americano*. Placemats are called *jogo Americano*, which means "American game." I don't really get that one, unless it alludes to those paper placemats in diners that let kids connect the dots and doodle.

Throughout the morning, more relatives and guests arrived. Jose had six siblings, three of whom had taken us under their wing during our other trips to Brazil. The siblings ranged in age from 24 to 52. Jose's parents had been married for 54 years, and his mother was 16 years old at the time of her marriage. One family member said it had been arranged, and another vehemently denied it. Her first child was born when she was 18, and her last child was born when she was 46. She and her husband were complete opposites. She was a chatterbox, always on the move; he preferred to observe with a broad, contagious smile.

For lunch, there were stone pots full of the ever-present *arroz e feijão* (rice and beans), chicken, a humongous hunk of pork, pureed red kidney beans resembling watery chocolate pudding, *salpicão* (a mixed dish with raisins, pitted olives, carrots, peas, corn, shredded chicken, and potato sticks; we had the choice of a bowl with or without mayo), okra swimming around in tan soupy liquid, *farofa* (kidney beans, pork, and some other ingredients mixed together with flour) and *tutu* (pureed kidney beans, sausage, and hard-boiled eggs, which Jim later described as "glue holding up sausages"). As soon as we put our forks down, we were encouraged to take second and third helpings. Of course, this is the custom in many cultures.

Sobremesa (dessert) consisted of blocks of *doce de leite* (kind of like caramel fudge), *flan*, something yellow in a bowl that looked like bread pudding, *broa* (like moist cornbread), *casserola* (like egg custard), and a giant bowl of figs marinated in a liquid that tasted like green gumdrops. Dessert was followed by another cup of heavily sugared, freshly hand-ground and put-through-a-flannel-sieve coffee.

Ehris

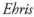

After lunch, Jose's brother, Sebastião, approached us. In Portuguese, he told us that he wanted to sell one of his horses and a mule. It turned out that the horse he was talking about used to belong to Jose, and was actually Jacques, whom I had ridden the year before. Until a few months before, when we bought the Gol, I had never purchased anything more expensive than a pair of shoes, but I did the negotiating for the horse and mule, since I was the most fluent in Portuguese. My dad stood there and did a lot of smiling. As an added bonus, Sebastião offered to throw in a 14-pound chicken. After a tough negotiation, we finally agreed upon a price for the horse and mule, and I even got delivery included.

The afternoon continued in the usual family holiday style with stories, jokes, gossip, and more coffee. Then began the farewells, identical to the greetings. Once again, my mom was bobbing and weaving like Sugar Ray Leonard. Jose's sister, Mariza, invited us to spend Easter at her house in Caratinga.

We drove off, with my mom asking Jose and Isabela countless questions, as usual.

CHAPTER TWENTY-NINE

Ehris

Living like pioneers lost its charm by week five. Our container was still making its journey across the Atlantic Ocean, so our house was empty (and I mean empty). The three of us were sleeping on the dark green air mattress, which my dad would pump up every night with Jose's compressor (the first night, he actually tried to inflate it with a blow dryer, but the plastic started to melt). Since we had no lamps, we would squish onto the pumped-up mattress when the sun went down, usually 8:00 P.M., and it would be totally deflated by dawn, leaving us sprawled on the brown tile floor. Since our only possessions were the things in our suitcases, which didn't include any comforts like sheets or blankets, we had been rolling up my sweatshirts for pillows.

Besides clothes, toiletries, a screwdriver, four white towels, the compressor, and the leaking air mattress, the only items we had while waiting for the container were one Polish stoneware bowl (which Mic had bought at Goodwill after we loaded the container in Connecticut), and an old fridge that came with the house. It wasn't frost-free, so every few days, we had to chisel ice out of the freezer with the screwdriver.

This period of minimalist existence was when we started playing the What-item-from-the-container-are-you-most-excited-to-see? game.

"The couch," I said, sitting cross-legged on the tile floor.

"It's between the washing machine and the dryer," my mom deliberated. "Because if I have to wash one more sweaty, muddy thing in the sink, then play around with those bamboo poles that hold up the clothesline, and then remember to get all the still-wet clothes off the line before the 4:00 rain...."

"The nail gun. Definitely the nail gun," my dad said wistfully.

Velya

Many Brazilians we met were convinced that everything was better in the United States. They apologized for Brazil's *favelas* (slums) and corrupt government. We assured them that the United States also had its share of problems, including poverty and corruption—they just hadn't heard about it. As Jim told them, our own Connecticut governor, John Rowland, had recently gone to prison for taking bribes! Ehris was getting sick of hearing me say, "It's too bad you can't take the best parts of the United States and the best parts of Brazil, and invent a whole new country." But it's true—all countries have their good and bad points.

"Jeem," Aureliano said over our staticky cell phone, "your container is stuck in port in Rio de Janeiro. They know 'bout the golf carts and chainsaws. They not gonna give you the container until you pay a bribe."

Brazil is a corruptocracy. If you want something done, you'll probably have to pay a bribe, and here's how you do it. After refusing, grumbling, complaining, and protesting, you suck it up and realize you have no choice if you want to rescue your hostaged possessions. As your wide-eyed 16-year-old daughter buckles her seatbelt, you check your lipstick in the rearview mirror of your gray VW Gol, and you try to not to dwell on the parenting books that advise, "Your child will follow your example, not your advice." Fully aware of the fact that what you're doing probably isn't legal, you begin your illicit drive to Banco do Brasil. After standing in one of Brazil's famously long bank queues—where customers commonly waste their entire lunch hour—you reluctantly deposit $3,000 U.S. into the bank account of an unscrupulous government worker. Adding insult to injury, you must send a fax to the account holder confirming that the bribe has been paid. There are no code words or secret phrases needed. "The $3,000 U.S. has been deposited into your account" finalizes the transaction.

That night, as I fought for my sliver of space on the leaky green air mattress, I thought about the horrible person I had become. In Connecticut, I had been a Brownie leader and a room mother, and conscientiously cut up those indestructible six-pack rings before throwing them in our recycling bin so ocean animals didn't suffer death by plastic. I had ignited young minds. Now, words like *payola, blackmail, kickback, hush money*, and *greased palms* described me—and if it meant that we'd soon have our queen-size TempurPedic bed with *sheets*, it was okay by me!

CHAPTER THIRTY

Ehris

"Yeah, I can do it," my mom answered when my dad asked if she and I could go buy 96 nuts and bolts for the *corral* gates. "All I really have to do is hold onto the steering wheel, right?"

Three days before, she had been trying to tighten the clothesline, and it had fallen on a Brazilian wasp nest the size of a volleyball. The outraged wasps had stung only her hands, which quickly blistered and oozed. They eventually looked exactly like E.T.'s—wrinkled, rubbery, and the color of mushroom gravy.

My dad, in his no dorkin' around way, got tired of waiting for Jose to send over the workers he had promised, so he started building the *corral* on his own. A *corral* in Brazil isn't a pen, like it is in the United States. It's a barn with no sides. My dad hired three guys who lived on our road, Edinho, Antonio, and Diego to help him.

A trip to *Ferreteria Castor* was nothing like making a quick stop at Home Depot. *Castor* means "beaver." Even though beavers don't exist in Brazil, there was a big, red, smiling, toothy one on their sign. One of the hardest cultural adjustments for us was how long it took to get anything accomplished. From buying coconuts to paying an electric bill, everything turned into a social occasion, and nobody was ever in a hurry.

At *Ferreteria Castor*, a bunch of drunk guys stood around the counter drinking *cachaça* out of an old hollowed-out wooden gourd. Complimentary *cachaça* was offered almost everywhere, including ice cream parlors, barber shops, and gas stations. As I counted out the 96 nuts and bolts, all the men tried to talk to my mom at once. She immediately became aware of just how pathetic her Portuguese was. Her foreign language skills were barely kindergarten-level, which was good, because there was a little girl at the hardware store. Their conversation (initiated by the kid) went like this: "Do you like peaches?"

"Yes, I like peaches."

"Do you like puppies?"

"Yes, I like puppies."

"Do you like carrots?"

"No, I do not like carrots."

Before we left the center of Ponte Nova, my mom said, "Ehris, why don't you turn on the cell phone just for a laugh, to see if anyone called us?"

I turned it on, and there was one urgent message from Aureliano, saying, "Jeem, this Aureliano. Your container is in Ponte Nova *right now*! The guy is at Esso gas station and he's wait for you to meet him so he can drive the truck to your farm."

"*What*? It's here *now*?" my mom shrieked. "We don't have any way to call Daddy and warn him!"

"We don't even know where the Esso station is!" I cried, and flagged down a kid on a moped for directions.

A 53-foot cargo container is actually the size of a tractor trailer, so it was pretty easy to spot once we found the Esso station. Since the driver was from Rio de Janeiro and didn't know the area, we agreed that he would follow us to our farm. He rumbled along at about three miles an hour, and had to stop along the way to move branches; avoid dogs, pregnant women, babies, and people with plaster casts; and chit-chat with neighbors he didn't even know.

My mom kept repeating, "Daddy is going to freak out when he sees this thing!"

We arrived at our farm about two minutes ahead of the truck. I hopped out and ran over to the *corral* where my dad was working alone, hammering together roof trusses. I shouted, "Daddy, the container is coming! *Right now!*"

He looked startled, but then regained his composure and came up with a plan. "Ehris, you and Mommy have to drive down the road and look for help! Stop anybody you see! Tell them we need help!"

My mom and I raced down the dusty road. We stopped at Antonio's house. I told Antonio, his wife Nair, and their grandson João Victor about our container, and asked if they knew anyone who could help. Antonio immediately volunteered, and 11-year-old João Victor got on the phone and implored neighbors in Portuguese, "The Americans need help! The Americans need help!"

Nair offered to help, but was wearing a plaster cast on her foot. There were a lot of things in Brazil we really couldn't figure out. White plaster casts were one of those things. Every day, my mom and I kept a tally of how many people we saw with these casts. In just one day, we counted 27 (for real!). The odd thing was that people only seemed to wear these casts for a few days, and then they were cut off. Nair, who said she broke her foot by falling off the doorstep when the baker delivered bread to their house, was cast-free and walking two days later.

Meanwhile, back at the farm, the truck driver and my dad were throwing clay roof tiles under the wheels to get the tractor trailer out of the mud. In between throwing the tiles and talking to the truck driver, my dad flagged down a guy driving a black motorcycle and tried to explain our problem. The guy didn't understand what my dad was saying (nobody ever did), but luckily, my mom and I were just returning from Antonio and Nair's house so I could translate.

When my dad opened the container, I thought our grandfather clock would fall out on top of him. Antonio, Nair, the motorcycle guy, two teenagers, the truck driver, and João Victor looked at the contents of the container in shock. So did we. Our surprise was due to the contrast of seeing our New England belongings in the palm-tree-lined clay driveway. I think the Brazilians were astonished by the enormity of what we owned.

Brazil is a country of contrasts. There's no middle class. Someone once told us, "In Brazil, everyone either *has* a maid, or *is* a maid." At our neighbors' homes, we were honored dinner guests. At Nair and Antonio's house, they insisted that we eat first. Then they washed our plates so *they* could eat. It wasn't like they had dishes that didn't match, or were chipped. These were the *only* plates they had. During the meal, bats swooped around in the rafters overhead. The following day, we were invited to an apartment in Belo Horizonte, and took an elevator to their penthouse. We ate a lavish lunch served by a uniformed maid. A nanny cared for the family's baby while we dined on quail eggs, mangoes, passion fruit, and *churrasco*.

The unloading process began. It took five hours. When we had loaded the truck on January 16th, it had been zero degrees and very windy. When we unloaded the truck on March 14th, it was 109 degrees.

The Brazilians were hard workers, and very interested in what we had brought (they weren't too thrilled about unloading the cumbersome stone benches, though). They had no idea what the sled or drill press were. João Victor, who came to our empty house every afternoon for English lessons and was the only Brazilian brave enough to pet Sylvia, ran toward me clutching a vibrating box.

"Oi, Ehriszinha!" he cried (all of our Brazilian friends called me *Ehriszinha*, "Little Ehris," as a term of endearment). *"Que é isso?"* I couldn't stop laughing. Somehow, my mom's battery-operated ultrasonic vibrating jewelry cleaner had turned on inside its box.

"Do you think it was vibrating all the way across the Atlantic Ocean?" my mom snorted. "Man, those are some pretty amazing batteries!"

Other than my parents' mattress getting wet, everything else had fared well. The contents of our four-bedroom Connecticut home didn't fit in our new two-bedroom house, so boxes were stacked to the ceiling in every room and spilled out onto the porch. Our helpers refused to accept any money, but asked if they could have the ratty blankets, rugs, and quilts we had used to cushion our furniture. I thought they planned to use them as dog beds or rags, but seeing my old pink dolphin quilt on João Victor's bed made me realize the unimportance of stuff. Stuff is just stuff. You can't enrich yourself with material possessions. However, as I learned from our neighbors, you *can* enrich yourself by offering love, kindness, and compassion.

With the simplest things, Nair made her corner of the world as beautiful as any queen's palace. We were invited to dinner at their house that night. Once again, the bats swooped overhead, but this time, our faded braided rug adorned the dirt floor. She handed me a bowl of stewed chicken feet to bring to the table and sagely told me, in Portuguese, "We may lack riches, but the greatest fortune is what lies in our hearts."

CHAPTER THIRTY-ONE

Velya

✻

Each of the animals reacted differently to their new home. Chauncey devoted all of his waking hours to sitting under a ramshackle lean-to. He would stare up at the clay roof, fixated on something we never saw. We began to call his hangout "Chauncey's clubhouse." Harry never caught his Brazilian mouse, but he spent his time stalking the six-foot-long lizards that lived on the hill under the papaya trees. Sylvia unknowingly terrified everyone who came to visit.

One morning, I noticed a bump on Sylvia's front elbow. Over the course of several days, the bump kept growing until it was the size of a tennis ball. Eventually, the bump developed a hole in the center. I forced myself to look inside and gagged when I saw that it was full of what appeared to be squirming maggot larvae. Ehris asked Guilherme to recommend a vet, but with a calm wave of his hand, he dismissively responded, "Nobody in Brazil goes to a vet. They treat these things themselves." We weren't calm about it. Neither was Sylvia.

Guilherme got us a carton of purple powder and a can of what looked like WD-40 to sprinkle and spray in Sylvia's worm-infested elbow. When I say purple, I mean purple like a grape Popsicle. Guilherme didn't warn us that the maggots would start wiggling, squirming, and dying as soon as the purple stuff hit them. Sylvia went *nuts* as hundreds of maggots began moving around and jumping out of her. We didn't know any of this was going to happen, so we did it indoors. Sylvia started leaping around the house, rubbing her elbow all over the white walls, leaving purple skid marks everywhere. Chauncey gobbled up the purple maggots that were writhing all over the tile floor.

It wasn't that Brazil was an unclean, dirty place. Worms, parasites, and bacteria thrive in tropical climates. We had those same issues in New England—it's just that our bitterly cold winters froze them before they could do much damage.

Revolting stuff had always fascinated me. When our pet canary, Clara, died, Jordan and I built her a tiny wooden coffin and held an elaborate funeral service for her. We buried her in the woods. Every day for about three weeks, I would dig up her coffin, pry off the lid, and check her state of decay. I don't think my mother had any idea I was doing this. Scientifically, the whole decomposition process fascinated me.

Instead of buying drumsticks, breasts, or thighs at the A&P, my mother bought whole chickens. By age ten, I was the one who got to cut them up, and I was entranced by how it all fit together—the ligaments and tendons, the soft mushy parts up near the chicken's spine, and the paper bag of organs inside the bird's carcass.

I suppose all of this was what made me an enthusiastic and memorable teacher. So, while Jim and Ehris dry-heaved at the sight of Sylvia's squiggling maggots, I ran for the camera. South America was offering me opportunities for countless new grossology lesson plans!

CHAPTER THIRTY-TWO

Velya

❀

Jose seemed distant and serious on the rare occasions we saw him after Carnaval. He made constant excuses as to why he couldn't ship the cows over to our farm, and why he hadn't built the *corral* or bought the milk tank. One day, Jim, Ehris, and I bumped into Guilherme in the narrow hallway of the internet café. Ehris made some small talk, since she was still the only one who could carry on a true conversation in Portuguese. As he was leaving, Guilherme turned and asked, "If you see Jose, can you remind him about the final payment on the farm?"

"*Como?*" Ehris questioned. Guilherme looked nervous. He said he had made a mistake and hurried off.

"What was that all about?" Jim asked Ehris, and she repeated the conversation. The blood drained from his face and he exhaled. "Let's go sit in the plaza."

We sat side by side on a concrete bench under a flowering *araribá* tree. Jim pulled a small purple notebook from his pocket, flipped through it, and said, "That was the final piece of the puzzle."

"*What* are you talking about?" I asked.

"Jose has been stealing from us," Jim said robotically. At that moment, Guilherme crossed the plaza, saw us, didn't make eye contact, and kept walking. A feeling of dread settled.

"What?" Ehris asked. She paused and added, "What's in the notebook?"

"Things just haven't been adding up, and I couldn't figure it out," Jim said. "We gave Jose more than enough money for the farm, the cows, the supplies to build the *corral*, and the milk tank. The way he's been avoiding me makes sense now."

I nervously asked, "Whaddya mean?"

"Now we know he never made the final payment on the farm," Jim said. "Who knows where the cows are, and what he did with all the other money."

Just then, our cell phone rang. Ehris answered. When the conversation ended, she looked at us and said, "That was Guilherme. He wants us to come to their apartment after lunch. He has something to tell us."

Jim nodded his head and predicted, "He wants to tell us what that son-of-a-bitch has been up to."

Shocked, I cried, "No way! Jose would never steal from us."

"He's like a member of the family," Ehris agreed. "He wouldn't do that." But as Jim showed us calculations in his purple notebook, it became clear that something was very wrong.

Despite the boys kicking tattered soccer balls, the guy peddling fragrant pineapples from the back of his pickup truck, the lady squeezing fresh sugarcane at a makeshift kiosk, and the kids milling around in blue and white parochial school uniforms, I had never felt so alone. It was as if the only three people left in the world were on that concrete bench 4,700 miles from Connecticut.

We took the elevator to Guilherme and Zoe's apartment. Zoe's swollen eyelids clearly indicated that she had been crying. Guilherme, normally animated and jolly, looked droopy and wilted. We all sat apprehensively in the living room. The real story poured out in Portuguese as Ehris translated.

Jose had told Guilherme that we were rich, entitled Americans who wanted to profit off of cheap Brazilian labor. He had asked Guilherme to inflate the price of his farm so he could lie about it to us. Then, we would send him more money, and Jose would pocket the difference. Guilherme had agreed, but once he got to know us, he realized we were *gente boa*, or good people, and felt ashamed by what he had done. Everyone was in tears. Zoe and Guilherme were grief-stricken that they had deceived us, and wanted to make things right. We assured them that we weren't mad at *them*, and thanked them for their honesty. Jim told Guilherme he'd had a feeling something was up, and that this confirmed his suspicions. With bowed head, he said, "I just didn't know how bad it actually was."

CHAPTER THIRTY-THREE

Ehris

Jose, the guy who'd helped me teach my eighth-grade chorus class the Portuguese words and bossa nova dance moves to "Girl from Ipanema," had coldheartedly swindled us. My dad tried to confront Jose, but he'd padlocked the gate at *Fazenda Granja do Bamba*, and never returned my dad's phone calls. The Brazilian lawyer had been all eager and convincing in the conference room, but had done nothing except cash my parents' check. We had no income, because Jose had stolen our herd of 200 cows. We didn't know who we could trust, and didn't know what Jose was involved in. After we decided that it was financially and emotionally impossible to stay in Brazil, the next two weeks were filled with heartbreaking and horrible tasks.

While my dad and Aureliano were at the Volkswagen dealership making arrangements with Luis to sell the Gol, 11-year-old João Victor came over for a final English lesson with my mom. From the field, I could see them on the *varanda*, surrounded by all the moving boxes and tearfully eating potato sticks. *Who eats potato sticks when they're upset?* I thought. In Connecticut, Ben & Jerry's right out of the carton would be comfort food. Cupcakes would be comfort food. But the only thing close to comfort food we had was potato sticks. *Brazilians and their potato sticks.* I smiled at the bittersweet memory of potato sticks on top of hot dogs, pizza, chicken fricassee, hamburgers, beef stroganoff, and potato salad, knowing that I'd never be able to eat them again once we left Brazil.

My job was to get a bridle on our mule, Jambi, so she'd be ready to go to her new farm when the horse trailer arrived. I kind of liked that I was the only one who could get close to her. Beautiful things shouldn't be tamed, or broken, or owned. I wasn't afraid of the wild that was in her. When she followed me without being asked and rubbed her head on mine, I felt my chest tighten up, and knew I was loved.

PART THREE

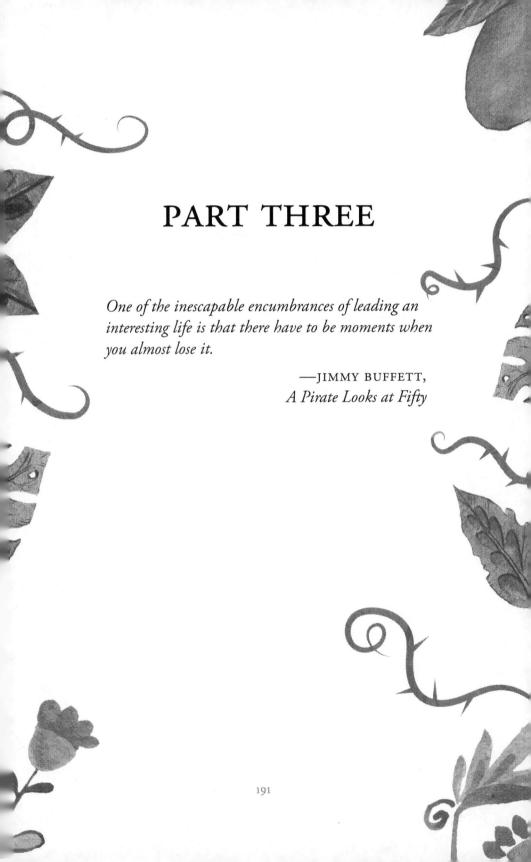

*One of the inescapable encumbrances of leading an
interesting life is that there have to be moments when
you almost lose it.*

—JIMMY BUFFETT,
A Pirate Looks at Fifty

CHAPTER THIRTY-FOUR

Ehris

We buried Sylvia in a beautiful spot overlooking the corral.

Her maggot issue cleared up and healed, but she developed autoimmune issues. We knew she'd never pass the vet inspection in São Paulo in order to bring her back to Connecticut.

"She'll become a street dog if we don't do it," my mom said, tears streaming down her face. "Even if her infections eventually clear up, nobody will be able to afford to feed her. These people barely have enough money to feed themselves, let alone a huge dog."

"Jose is taking everything from us," I sobbed. "Even Sylvia."

I fed Sylvia an entire package of *Passatempo* cookies while my dad and Antonio dug her grave. We sat with her and waited for my mom to come back to the farm with the vet. The somber vet was rattled because he had never put a dog to sleep before. It just wasn't done in rural Brazil. They shot them, or let them become street dogs. My dad knelt, and with a catch in his throat, whispered, "You're such a good pup, Sylvia." Even craggy Antonio cried as the vet gave her the injection. With all of us petting her, Sylvia died with her head in my mom's lap.

CHAPTER THIRTY-FIVE

Velya

We gave Aureliano both of our golf carts. Knowing that his kids would love driving them as much as Mic and Ehris had brought me a little happiness. Jim gave the chainsaws, weed whackers, nail guns, and generator to our grateful neighbors. Guilherme was going to try to sell our farm after we left Brazil, and we didn't want Jose to get wind of what was going on, so we had to lie to our neighbors and tell them we were leaving Brazil because of my mother's declining health. They were openly weeping the day they helped us load the cargo container, as were we.

The cast iron frying pans from TJ Maxx left me with a bittersweet memory. On the day we left Brazil, Jim gave them to solemn Diego, who had helped build the *corral*. He accepted them as if they were gold bricks. At sunset from the *varanda*, we watched Diego head home, trudging up the hill behind our farm with the three frying pans on his head. Our dream was dead.

CHAPTER THIRTY-SIX

Velya

❁

With the little money we had left, even though we had
paid Jose in full for our farm, we paid Guilherme the
final amount he was owed.

After only two months in Brazil, we returned to
Connecticut. We no longer had a house, or jobs, or dreams,
or goals, or money. Trust can take years to build, but only
seconds to break. The monetary loss was horrible, but the
betrayal was far worse. Betrayal makes you feel dead inside.
Betrayal shatters you and makes you wonder about things
like monkey socks. Betrayal changes everything. When we'd
hugged on that mountaintop and his whiskers scratched my
cheek, Jose had already betrayed us. The mistake was ours,
for trusting him.

During the nine-hour plane ride back to the United
States, Jim stared out the window and said only one thing.
"It's probably a good thing I didn't see Jose after we found out
what he did to us. I think I would've killed him."

Vivian and Jeff took us in, and for six weeks, we holed
up in their house and licked our wounds. Then we began the
detached, obligatory process of rebuilding our lives. The only

thing that made me feel a little bit better was something Jeff had said when he picked us up at Newark Airport: "If someone really wants to steal from you, they're going to figure out a way to do it. There's nothing you can do to stop them."

CHAPTER THIRTY-SEVEN

Velya

❁

My mother hurriedly met Jim and me at their front door. She gave me the covert nod to join her in the bathroom before I even had a chance to speak. My mother always beckoned me to the pantry or bathroom when she wanted to confide in me with my father out of earshot.

"Mom, what's going on here?" I asked, examining the bruises on her forehead, under her eyes, and down her shoulder. The angry purple shade would have been royal if it had been on her sleeve instead of her skin. Except for the sickly yellow, the colors in the bruises reminded me of the striations of an amazing sunset. Absurdly, the adage she had taught me as a child, *red sky at morning, sailors take warning,* popped into my head, and I pushed it way.

"I can't tell you. That wouldn't be fair to him," my mother pleaded.

I spluttered, "Fair to *him*? You mean *Daddy* did this?!" I had to close my eyes so the room would stop spinning.

"I can handle Daddy. This wasn't all his fault. It's a very complicated story."

"You call *this* handling Daddy? Tell me the complicated story," I said, knowing I had to document the bruises. I rummaged through my purse for my camera—the camera I had brought to show her photos of Brazil, not to photograph black and blue marks.

"He was going around all day swearing, swearing, swearing and I told him to stop. He was calling me every imaginable thing under the sun. Then I get confused if it was a dream, or if it was really me," she started to babble, "because then I'm a young girl in a car…I don't think we were even married yet, and I *think* we were in a car…I think we had just left a dance, and he was calling me a drunken slut, and you know I don't smoke or drink…and then I was in a car, and he was hitting me, and then I remember his face looking at me. I hate it. I just want peace. You were gone…in Brazil…and he was swearing all day, and I told him to stop and we got into a fight." She squinted at me and made boxing motions like Muhammad Ali.

"A fight?" I asked incredulously, eyebrows raised and eyes wide open.

"Yes, we started fighting," she repeated, and once again made the boxing motions.

"Mom, you can't stay here like this! One of you has to go," I begged. "We've told you this before. You can leave with us now, or we can have Daddy leave. Jim's out there with him in the living room."

In disbelief, she asked, "You mean leave *now*? No, I couldn't do that to him. Not today. I have to talk to him first. I can't just leave. If I do, he'll kill himself. I can't leave the house. That's what he wants."

"Mom, nothing's going to happen to the house. He can't sell the house. We won't let that happen," I promised.

"He'll rip up all my books and throw everything of mine outside!" she exclaimed.

"That's not going to happen, Mom. And most important, if you don't care about yourself, how about what this is doing to me, and even more important, think about your granddaughter. Think about Ehris. What kind of respect is she going to have for you as a woman if you don't do something about this?" I implored.

I knew my mother wasn't listening as she continued, "You know, I wear these Depends and sometimes the poop leaks out."

"Yeah, so that can happen," I shrugged. "What's the big deal?"

She continued, "He started yelling, 'There's shit all over the goddamn house. Shit! Shit! Shit! All I ever do is clean up shit!'"

I dropped onto the closed toilet seat in my parents' bathroom. My brain felt as if it were dissolving and dripping out of my ears. We had been back from Brazil for seven days. Everything we owned was in a cargo container somewhere on the Atlantic Ocean. We had been gone for such a short time, and *this* was what I had come home to? How long had this been going on? I thought about some incidents that had taken place in the months leading up to our move to Brazil.

One of my mother's many revolving-door home health aides had pulled me aside in the kitchen to complain about my father. "He was so mad that the veins were popping out of his head! I thought he was gonna have a stroke," she divulged, "but, honey, nobody calls me a nigger! And he better not pull that shit ever again!" I had encouraged her to walk out, to quit, yet I knew how desperately she needed the money.

The aides had constantly confided in me with reports about what was happening in my parents' home. One live-in aide said, "I don't know who the patient is around here, your father or your mother. Do you know that man pounded on the bathroom door this morning because I was taking too long in the shower? Nobody pounds on *my* bathroom door!"

A different aide had grumbled, "Why in god's name does your father have to leave the house at 5:30 in the morning to go swim his laps? That old fool expects me to be up, dressed, and gettin' your mother ready for the day by the time he leaves. It's still dark at 5:30 in the morning!"

My racing mind returned to the incomprehensible scene before me in the bathroom. I stood up and guided my mother to the living room. "Dad, what's going on here?" I asked non-combatively. "Do you know anything about these bruises?"

My father exploded with rage. His face turned from red to purple. Veins throbbed on his forehead and in his neck. He furiously spit out, "I'm disowning you!" Turning to my mother before storming out the door he announced, "You have to decide between Velya and me, and you have to decide now!"

I helped my mother back to the bathroom and pulled down her elastic waist pants, and then her Depends. She faced me as I guided her hands to the arms of the commode chair, keeping a hand on her rounded back as she eased her body down onto the white plastic seat. Her knee made an ungodly grinding sound, and she smelled faintly like old dollar bills.

As a little girl, after my mother lifted me from the bathtub, I used to stand on this same toilet seat as she briskly dried me with a soft towel. With my face pressed into her chest, she'd always say the exact same thing: "Now you're gonna feel like a million bucks!"

A couple days before, I had given Chauncey, still full of Brazilian dust, a much-needed bath in Vivian and Jeff's kitchen sink, and caught myself saying it, too. *No*, I'd assured myself, *I'm not becoming my mother*.

I looked out the bathroom window and saw a new family of Mallard ducks on the lake. The brown-headed mother, drab in comparison with her green-headed mate, quacked at a duckling gone astray. Jordan said that for a long time, he'd only been having non-confrontational conversations with our parents—it was safer that way, for everyone. He called them: *So, how many swans are on the lake?* conversations.

When I handed my mother some toilet paper, she said exactly what I expected her to say, because I had heard it all before. "We can manage just the way it is. We'll be fine. It will be okay. I can handle Daddy."

But this time it wasn't fine. Something in me had broken.

CHAPTER THIRTY-EIGHT

Ehris

When people say that growing up can happen overnight, they're wrong. It can happen in an instant. For me, that instant was on a park bench in Brazil.

"How could Jose have done that to Daddy, who did so much for him?" I blubbered.

"I don't know, Ehris. Obviously, I can't stop thinking about it," my mom said vacantly. "I wonder if he got involved with drugs, or another woman...."

"What happened to *Jeem, I do for you like you do for me?*" I mocked. "All we wanted to do was try something new and live on a farm. How can people do that to each other?"

There were times after Brazil when I was worried about myself, and I actually Googled "dissociative amnesia." There were big chunks of time that I didn't remember. I guess it's all buried in my brain somewhere.

Memory loss is a way of coping with damage. It's strange. It's like getting to the theater halfway through the movie. You know you've missed something—you just don't know if it's important. So, you try to lose yourself in the story, and hope the gaps don't matter. Maybe it's totally fine not to know what you've missed.

We don't just forget things because they don't matter. We also forget things because they matter too much. Why do I remember the white kitchen ceiling fan at the rental house, but have no memory of leaving Vivian and Jeff's house and moving there? The blades of the ceiling fan were battle-scarred, and so were the doors of the kitchen cabinets. Even as messed up as all of us were, we laughed every time we forgot that you couldn't open the cupboards while the stupid fan was on, because the blades *whack, whack, whacked* the doors.

I know I worked at the Bank Street Coffee House for a year and a half, but I don't remember the months I must have spent finishing high school online. Why can I picture the mouse family jumping out of the engine when my dad started up the lawnmower at the rental house, but I have no idea how all the stuff from our cargo container got unloaded and stored in our friend Jacqui's basement? I remember the pizza delivery guy conking his head on the icy driveway and passing out, and the way the house shook when Mic backed my dad's construction van through the garage door, but I don't remember my dad having any interest in life.

"That's it," he said all the time now. "We can never trust anyone ever again." My dad wasn't the man he used to be. He had lost his gentle side. The bags under his eyes broke my heart, but he kept everything to himself. He went through the motions of life but spoke very little. One weekend, we actually kept track, and he spoke a total of four sentences. We were polite and careful with him, but he just sat in the bluish flicker of the TV and watched mindless junk. I had no idea what he was thinking about as he sagged on the couch with his hand over his eyes. He went to work. He came home.

He was there, but he wasn't. Jose had been like a brother. Betrayal doesn't just change relationships. It changes people.

My dad saved us from financial ruin by resurrecting Urban Crossroads. He rose before sunrise, worked 12 hour days, and did estimates late at night and on weekends. He had become a zombie, but never complained. He just did what had to be done.

We were in the furnished rental house on a month-to-month basis because we had no idea where we would end up. My mom was sending out resumes all over the United States for my dad, who planned to return to the corporate world. She decided to take the advice of her teacher friends, who had urged her to "take her show on the road." She created *How Cool Is That?! Hands-On Science* and began teaching classes like *Alka-Seltzer Rockets* and *Bungee Jump Barbie* in an effort to make back some of the money Jose had stolen. I was a commuting freshman at Western Connecticut State University, majoring in Anthropology/Sociology. Mic was still in school at the University of Puerto Rico, and slept on the rental house couch when he was home for the summer.

I don't know why I felt the need to punish myself, but for the 18 months that we lived in that house, I refused to let my dad get my mattress out of Jacqui's basement. I stood firm about sleeping on a striped yoga mat. Punishing myself for Jose's wrongs made about as much sense as a Kamikaze pilot wearing a crash helmet.

CHAPTER THIRTY-NINE

Ehris

"I loved him so much," Nazey said faintly.

"Loved *who* so much?" my mom asked, perched on the end of the hospital bed.

"Your brother," she responded.

"My *brother*?" Confused, my mom questioned, "Why are you talking about him in the past tense?"

"Who is your brother?"

"Jordan," my mom prodded, looking perplexed.

"No, not him." Nazey closed her eyes as if it would help her think. "I love him, but not him." A nurse came in to take Nazey's temperature and check her IV bag. She was still kind of out of it from her aortic valve replacement anesthesia. As usual, my mom and I were at her side as she recovered. I felt like I shouldn't interrupt the conversation. It felt like something important was in the air.

"Do you mean *your* brother?" my mom offered.

"Who's that?" Nazey responded weakly.

"Chuck," my mom said.

Nazey eagerly exclaimed with recognition, "Yes, yes!

Chuck!" My mom and I gave each other puzzled looks, which Nazey didn't notice. She slowly scanned the room and asked my mom, "Where's Daddy?"

"He went to get an oil change and emissions inspection on the car," my mom explained. "He won't be back for a while."

With that, Nazey pushed the controls to raise the hospital bed to an upright position. With more strength, she studied my mom and said, "Chuck came to our house when you were just babies. He was having trouble with his wife."

My mom said, "Yeah, I kind of remember when he came. Wasn't his wife's name Rose?"

Nazey cocked her head. "How do you remember that? You weren't even in kindergarten yet."

"I can picture her face. I remember her sitting in the dining room."

"He came to see me," Nazey said shakily. "He needed me, and I let him down."

"What do you mean?" my mom asked. "I always had a feeling something bad happened between you two."

I knew that Nazey hadn't seen Chuck for over 40 years, and didn't know his whereabouts. I also knew that ever since my mom and Uncle Jordan were little kids, the Chuck topic had not been open for discussion. Nazey didn't know that my mom had been searching for Chuck online for almost 20 years, with no success.

"He was having marriage problems, and he was trying to decide whether to try again with Rose," Nazey said, wiping at her eyes with the Kleenex I handed her. "We talked for a long, long time, and I told him he should call her. The problem was Daddy. He wanted to know why Chuck was here, how long he was staying, when he was leaving, what did he want...."

My mom cut her off. "Yup, that sounds like Daddy."

"Then I did something I never, never should have done," Nazey confessed. "Chuck used the phone in the foyer to call Rose. I should have known...he was a radio man in the Navy...he heard the click...he heard the click...I should have known...I should have known...I shouldn't have done it...."

"Done what?" my mom urged.

"I went down to the patio where we had the outside phone."

"Oh, yeah!" my mom said, nodding her head. "I forgot about that phone."

"I picked up the receiver and listened in on his call. I heard Rose say he needed a mother, and she wasn't going to be his mother. I had to know...I had to know. Daddy was making me crazy about why he was there and when he was leaving. When Chuck got off the phone, he came down to the lake where I was playing with you two, and asked if there was another phone in the house because he had heard a click. I told him that was the only phone. Then, the outside phone rang and he knew...he knew...he knew...and he got this look on his face...I'll never forget the look...and he said he was leaving. I never saw him again."

My mom and I sat in stunned silence for a moment.

My mom responded reassuringly, "Well, Mom, I'm glad you finally told me. I always thought something had happened. You shouldn't blame yourself. You had to keep peace with Daddy because you didn't want us to come from a broken home, like you did. The person you should blame, and you never have, is your mother."

I don't know if Nazey was aware that we were still in the room as she continued, trance-like. "I called him, and he never called me back. I wrote to him, and he never answered my letters. That's why I can't go sit on the patio. I see that phone…I see that phone…."

I held Nazey's hand. My mom stroked her arm and said, "I always kind of wondered why that phone just disappeared. Mom, what you did probably wasn't the smartest thing, but you're blaming the wrong people. I think your mother screwed up Chuck more than she screwed you up. He was practically a baby when she left, and nobody even knows *why* she left. And what was Daddy's problem? What difference did it make how long Chuck stayed, or why he was there? He was your *brother*, for god's sake!"

"You shouldn't blame yourself, Nazey," I said.

Nazey rallied to instruct my mom, "I need you to write to Rose and explain all of this. I want to, but I'm embarrassed. Look in the top dresser drawer in your old room. There's an envelope where I wrote *Rose, Rose, Rose,* and circled it. I can't write to her."

"You know her *address?*" my mom asked in disbelief.

"She wrote to me and told me Chuck had died."

"Chuck is *dead?*" My mom looked and sounded shocked. "How come nobody ever told me? When did he die?"

"He died in 1990. I couldn't tell you. I couldn't."

"He's been dead for *19 years?*" my mom asked in disbelief.

"I didn't know he had died until Rose sent me a letter last year," Nazey said, starting to shut down.

"Okay, okay, I'll write to her and explain it all. Don't worry," my mom assured her. "I'm really proud of you for telling us all this, Mom. You did what you had to do for your children. You didn't want what happened to you and Chuck to happen to us. I understand."

"I want you to go to the house and find the two cameos. Look in the black velvet box in the bottom drawer of my dresser."

"The cameos Chuck bought you in Italy when he was in the war?" my mom asked.

"Yes. Daddy always wanted me to get them made into pendants, but I couldn't...I couldn't...."

"Okay, I'll get them. Do you want me to give one to Jordan?" my mom asked.

"Yes."

"Do you want me to tell him about Chuck?" my mom asked.

"Yes."

"But you don't want me to tell Daddy, right?" my mom confirmed.

"Right."

"I'll write to Rose and explain everything. But Mom, it wasn't your fault. You shouldn't blame yourself. If Chuck let something stupid like that come between you two, he must have been really messed up. I'll write to Rose."

Nothing weighs so heavily as a secret, and some are only to be told to daughters and granddaughters. After revealing her 47-year secret, Nazey started to slip out of who she was. She shed everything, the way a snake discards its skin. I think Nazey had always hoped to reconcile with her brother, but once she learned he had been dead for almost two decades, she began preparing to leave for good. This was the last time we connected cognitively with her. She closed up as tightly as the little black velvet box that held the two Italian cameos.

CHAPTER FORTY

Velya

❖

Jordan and I were ushered into a conference room at the law office of Ann Crowley-Foster, and settled our mother. She asked for the Kleenex she always palmed now, and we found a wadded-up one in the pocket of her royal blue fleece jacket. Sometimes, we found it up her sleeve, old-lady style, like a tricky magician.

Jordan had arranged this meeting so our mother could speak freely to her attorney—the new attorney our parents now shared. Freely, meaning our father was not there to put words in her mouth or monitor her conversation. He thought Jordan had taken her to Mill Plain Diner for breakfast. He had no idea where we really were.

Our father was trying desperately to put our mother in a nursing home. She wanted to remain in the place she'd lived since 1960. Jordan and I knew it was just a matter of time before our father had his way, as he now held her ill-gotten power-of-attorney. Our mother had clearly reached the point of being incapable of understanding what she was doing when she had rescinded the previously-held power from us, and given it to our father. Ann Crowley-Foster had drawn up the paperwork and witnessed the change, without our knowledge.

Our father had actually told Jordan that our mother's declining health was "cramping his style," and he wanted "to have her put away." Jordan and I wanted her wishes to be heard by someone besides us—to be heard by someone with power and authority—before it was too late. Ann Crowley-Foster said the holder of a power of attorney is obligated to honor the wishes of the grantor. We wanted our mother's wishes clearly known.

After selecting our own spots around the rectangular laminate table and making awkward small talk about the glorious October morning, Jordan swiveled his seat and asked, "Mom, what would it do to you if someone told you, 'You have to leave the house?'"

In a quavering voice, she responded, "It would kill me."

The lawyer leaned forward in her rolling chair, making sure she had heard correctly. She looked into our mother's eyes and quietly asked, "Why don't you want to leave the house?"

Our mother looked at the lawyer as if she were missing the most obvious of answers. She looked at her as if she had asked, "Do you plan on doing any blinking today?"

There was only one answer. She clearly stated, "It is where I want to be."

The dysfunctional marriage of our parents had made it necessary for Jordan and me to take sides. We had tried everything not to be in that law office, but for our parents' entire marriage, our father had attempted to control every aspect of our mother's life. She repeatedly told us, "I have never had a true discussion with that man."

The attorney concluded the meeting by saying, "I will have to report everything that went on here to your father."

I saw the writing on the wall, and slipped the photos of our black-and-blue mother across the laminate table to Ann Crowley-Foster, who glanced down at them without actually touching them.

"Do you report all of our *father's* conversations with you to our *mother*?" I asked.

She ushered us to the door, and I knew she would be calling our father.

Exactly one month after our visit to the lawyer, the power of attorney she had entrusted to our father was used to admit our mother to Laurel Ridge Nursing Home. Neither Jordan nor I knew what had really gone on.

We did know that Ann Crowley-Foster had recommended that a social worker go to the house for an assessment. According to my father, my mother was going crazy when she got there. The social worker claimed she was yelling, "They want to kill me!" These were the words she had used to describe what it would do to her if she had to leave her home. I suspect my father had spent the day goading her with his usual taunts about selling "the goddamn house," and her being unable to even wipe her own "goddamn ass," and that the woman who was coming over was going to "commit" her.

My father claimed she was going berserk. My mother's aide later told Jordan, "She was fine. Your mother was a sweet lady, and never gave me no problems." An ambulance took her to the emergency room, and she went directly to Laurel Ridge from there. My father and I were no longer speaking. Jordan was at a music studio in Woodstock, New York. After recording a song ironically entitled "Love, Peace, and Freedom," he checked his voicemail and heard a terse, "I committed your mother to Laurel Ridge today."

I learned you can just stop loving someone—as simple as that.

CHAPTER FORTY-ONE

Velya

For many reasons, I found it extremely difficult to visit my mother at Laurel Ridge Nursing Home. She didn't want to be there, Jordan and I didn't want her to be there, and every single time we saw her, she asked, "Oh, are you here to take me home?" She'd beg, "If you just wheel me down to the front desk, I can make arrangements for them to send me home."

If I'd had my way, I would have done just that. As disgusted as I was with my father, I just couldn't bring myself to hurt my mother by telling the truth: "Daddy won't let you come home." When you love someone, you don't want to be the one who brings their world shattering down around them.

I also had issues with the word *visit*. The dictionary defines *visit* as "go to see a place, as for entertainment." There is absolutely nothing entertaining about going to, or living in, a nursing home. I held my tears hostage when Jordan and I found our mother slumped over in her wheelchair, seated around a large table with other slumped-over patients. At the head of the table, an animated woman with marmalade-colored hair and a candy-apple-red twin set read aloud to the group from *The Ridgefield Press*, the local newspaper. She seemed oblivious to all the slumping.

At the end of the visit, as we were leaving, our mother asked brightly, "Oh, are you going to bring the car around to the front entrance?" As my eyes filled with tears, Jordan tried to make me laugh by unzipping his jacket and flashing me the inside breast pocket, bulging with pilfered purple latex gloves.

"I wear them when I pump gas," he explained. "I like to think of them as my 'lovely parting gifts,' courtesy of Laurel Ridge."

CHAPTER FORTY-TWO

Velya

After my mother had been at Laurel Ridge for a year, I hoped my father would come to his senses and bring her home. He was spending over $12,000 a *month* out of pocket to keep her there. Twenty-four-hour home care would have cost half that amount. As angry as we were with our father, both Jordan and I had ambivalent feelings about our mother. Her life was the sum of all her choices, and those choices included never standing up to—or confronting—our father. So many times over the years, we had encouraged her to leave him, to take a stand, to come and live with Jim and me. Jordan would become enraged when our mother said, "You don't understand. I can't leave him. It's a generational thing."

She wouldn't stand up to our father, and in holding her power of attorney, he also held all the cards. We were powerless to help her, and told ourselves that at least she was warm, safe, and fed at Laurel Ridge. Months went by, and as I slowly began to recover from our Brazilian betrayal, I finally felt strong enough to take on my father. Thanks to Jim's hard work, we had saved enough money to buy a house. It was actually Jim's idea for me to petition to become my mother's conservator. Since my father wouldn't let her come home, we wanted to do the next best thing and have my mother, and a full-time aide, come live with Jim and me. Since our father held the power of attorney, we knew it would be a long shot, but Jordan and I decided we would try one last time to help our mother.

"If we lose this battle, at least we'll know we tried," Jordan said. "Whatever happens, I'll be able to look at myself in the mirror."

I agreed. The paperwork was filed, and we prepared our case for probate court. Jordan and I visited our mother at the nursing home. To strengthen our claim, we videotaped her telling us how much she wanted to leave Laurel Ridge and move in with Jim and me, if she couldn't go home to Ridgefield. Like kidnappers, we had her hold that day's newspaper to prove the video was current. Off-camera, and as part of the normal conversation we were having with her, she haltingly defined *faux pas*, slowly spelled *loquacious*, and told us how much she loved us.

During all of this, I discovered an old house for sale in Woodbury, Connecticut. Jim and I agreed that I would take a drive over to see it rather than waste our realtor's time by scheduling a showing. We had always been fascinated by historic homes, and by the fact that when people walk into them, they don't automatically know where the bathroom is. When I pulled into the driveway, I kicked myself for having passed over the house so many times on Realtor.com. It looked nothing like the blurry online photos. Before I even climbed out of the car, I knew this was the one.

It was a simple square Connecticut farmhouse, added onto many times over the years. At the far end of the property, a meadow turned to pinewoods. Potentially lethal icicles, some of them six feet long, hung from the roof like the frozen teeth of a Tyrannosaurus Rex. Winter had been especially rough that year. The piles of snow surrounding the house were so high, they gave me the perfect vantage point to peer in the six-over-six windows. The frost on them was like bits of lace. The kitchen walls had appeared SpongeBob-yellow in the listing photos, but they were actually a traditional mustard color. Wide board floors with wrought-head nails ran throughout the first floor. The early American fireplace had a massive hearth. It was surrounded by a wall of raised paneling, where someone had hung a wreath of dried hydrangeas I planned to take down as soon as we moved in. I could have sworn the house whispered to me.

"Wait until you see this place! It's perfect," I chattered to Jim from my cell phone. "It's empty, and really old, and just past that farm that sells the free-range eggs. Those crummy photos don't do it justice. Let's see if Suzanne can get us inside tonight to see it. You're going to love this house," I promised.

To myself I said, *this is the place. This is where we can finally heal.*

Once inside, I saw it had a downstairs back bedroom and a nearby bathroom that would be perfect for my mother. There was a lovely guest room for the aide, and the wide hallways would perfectly accommodate my mother's wheelchair or walker. Our lawyer of 28 years was working simultaneously on two legal issues for us: my conservatorship and the house closing.

The day after appearing in probate court, Jim and I closed on the new house. We were close friends with both the realtor and the lawyer, and spent much of the closing discussing the court proceedings and speculating on the outcome, which would be ruled upon within a week.

CHAPTER FORTY-THREE

Velya

❀

Old houses groan, and creak, and sigh, but if you tune them out a bit, you can ignore the theatrics. They speak to you, if they want to—sometimes in whispers, a bit at a time. If you're open to hearing what the lives within the walls have to say, the rewards can be transformative. Old houses are for those who can tolerate a little imperfection in their living, and owning one is kind of like knowing a really great secret.

The 12-room house was in foreclosure, and had been vacant for five years as the asking price dropped and dropped. When the bank accepted our lowball offer, Jim arranged for 11 men, most of them Brazilians who worked with him in his construction business, to help us on the day of the move. I thought I had mentally allocated a place in the house for all of our belongings.

Jim posted me in the garage, as I was supposed to direct the men where to go with each box or piece of furniture. When the first things off the moving truck were saddles, bridles, reins, and a huge box labeled *cow medicine and calf nipples*, I realized I'd forgotten about at least half of our possessions. I had approximately three seconds to decide where each box was supposed to go, and didn't even know what we were calling many of the rooms in the new house. Men speaking Portuguese wandered aimlessly, looking for logical places to put their boxes. One narrow staircase was completely blocked by our queen-sized TempurPedic bed. An older guy I had never seen before carried a cardboard box labeled *Veal's bras* as if it held holy relics. He kind of bowed to me as I pointed him in the direction of our bedroom. Ehris insisted we save the box I had neurotically labeled *doilies, or however you spell it* to remind her of the nightmare of packing with me—the me I used to be. When it was all over, hardly any of our things wound up where they were supposed to, but eating pizza with all the men at our long-lost dining room table was a wonderful feeling. We were home.

CHAPTER FORTY-FOUR

Velya

I received the probate court ruling by mail about a week later. It took several days for me to compose a letter, which Jordan and I both signed, to the court-appointed attorney who had met with my mother for 30 minutes.

Dear Attorney Brennan:

The judge has issued his ruling, and our mother, Neysa Jancz, will spend the rest of her life in an institution. She will probably never see the 12-room home in Woodbury, Connecticut where she could have lived her final years surrounded by family, the classical music she adores, books, teenagers coming and going, and cats settling on her lap. She won't hear a washing machine on its spin cycle, won't smell lasagna in the oven, won't see her beloved daughter on a daily basis or sit outdoors on a lovely stone patio. She'll be "walked" (yes, that's the actual term they use) at Laurel Ridge, but there won't be any trips to the grocery store, the movies, or a simple ride in a car.

As our mother's court-appointed attorney, you held a tremendous responsibility, and you dropped the ball because you chose not to see Neysa Jancz—the real Neysa Jancz. You made no inquiries as to why she is in the situation she is. Yes, you examined the Laurel Ridge visitor's book and saw that our father visits every day, as he should; for jailers see their prisoners on a daily basis. Yet did you also explore the fact that our mother does not talk to our father when he visits? In court, you spoke of their long marriage. Did you know our mother removed her wedding ring when our father "committed" her (his word) to Laurel Ridge, and will not put it back on? Had you asked, we could have told you that our mother slipped tranquilizers into our father's coffee on a nightly basis in order to make life with him bearable.

I was disowned by my father because I questioned him about severe bruising on my mother's face and shoulder, after a private conversation with my mother in her bathroom while she still lived at 171 Mountain Road. My mother permitted me to take photos of the bruises. Were you aware of this fact?

Our mother has told anyone who will listen, including her attorney, who was in the courtroom, and our father, who holds her power of attorney, that she wants to live and die in the house she has occupied since 1960. When do a person's wishes stop being their wishes?

You chose to focus on the fact that Neysa Jancz's bills are being paid and she is being fed. "Three hots and a cot" came to mind when you introduced this line of questioning. Is this the best our mother can hope for? A woman who worked hard her entire life and invested wisely—do you even know where she worked or what she did? Is it fair that the money she earned and saved is being used to keep her in a place she doesn't want to be? Didn't you wonder why two children and their respective spouses would try so hard to get their mother out of an institution?

It's too late now for our mother. Our only hope is our father dies first, and we can then legally remove her from

Laurel Ridge and bring her home. I'd like you to think about our mother the next time you become someone's court-appointed attorney. Three sides—there are always three sides to every story. Her side, his side, and the truth. Until you're willing to examine all three of those sides and then *make your decision, you are not doing your job.*

Sincerely yours,
Velya Jancz-Urban
Jordan Jancz

I sent a copy of the letter to the probate judge, too. I got a note back from his secretary informing me it was "inappropriate to send such a letter to the court." I wanted to scream, "I sent it to a *man*, not a *court!*"

CHAPTER FORTY-FIVE

Velya

❉

In the weeks following the judge's ruling, I did two things. I avoided the back bedroom that would have been my mother's, and let it become a dumping ground for unopened boxes and anything I didn't know what to do with. I robotically sorted through our belongings. I decorated, numbly filled closets, hung mirrors and paintings, brought empty cardboard boxes to the dump—but couldn't let myself love the house.

The second thing I did was dream about my father—violent, vivid nightmares where I punched him in the head and screamed at him. I clearly remember one dream where I rhythmically slapped him in the face and shouted, "What (slap) is (slap) wrong (slap) with (slap) you? How (slap) could (slap) you (slap) do (slap) this (slap) to (slap) her?" His head rocked back and forth with each blow, and it was very satisfying to hurt him.

I also had two recurring dreams. As the writer, producer, director, and star of all my dreams, I knew I was sending myself messages.

In one dream, I was always naked and in need of a 32-ounce container of Stonyfield vanilla yogurt. I told myself if I just stayed on course in the grocery store and headed only to the dairy department, and didn't get sidetracked or make eye contact, then nobody would even notice my nakedness. I saw myself doing this, and knew I was stark naked, and knew all the customers knew I was naked, but they didn't say anything. I liked to think of it as an *Emperor's New Clothes* dream all wrapped up in deception and trust issues.

Another dream involved me constantly forgetting to nurse a baby that wasn't mine, but I was somehow responsible for it. My breasts were rock hard, engorged, and eventually leaking all over the place, but I'd see the baby in a corner and forget about feeding it. A few days would go by, and I'd think, "Wait a minute. Did I ever feed that baby?" And still, I made no move to do so.

Even an amateur would be able to interpret the insights of these dreams. I was forced to bear the consequences for my failure to perform as expected. Clearly, babies represent our vulnerability over some situations in our lives, and could breasts be a more obvious symbol of mothering, love, and protection?

Ehris

I saw Jose as two different people. I was furious that he had robbed my parents, ruined everything we had worked for, and destroyed my dad's spirit. But I missed the Jose who couldn't finish a joke without laughing, who had urged me to sample Brazilian foods like *jabuticaba* and *carambola* with "Try, Ehris, try!" and "I'm a love this stuff!" I missed his stories.

Anything could turn into a funny story with Jose. Brazilians pride themselves on dressing well. The Brazilians we met would never leave the house in pajama pants and slippers, or wear ripped, stained, or un-ironed clothes. When we stayed at Jose and Isabela's house, we all felt bad about giving our dirty laundry to Fatima, but they insisted. One day, I left my wet bathing suit hanging in the bathroom to dry. Fatima washed *and* somehow ironed it (I have no idea how you iron a bathing suit without melting it). Brazilians iron washcloths, sheets, dishtowels, jeans, and t-shirts. Clothing is a big deal in Brazil. There's a genuine desire and importance to always look your best.

One morning, Jose made a very early trip to the airport, which was three hours away in Belo Horizonte, to drop off a friend. I was lying in a hammock on the *varanda* when Jose got back, and slyly looked him up and down. He had on a form fitting short-sleeved red shirt with side slits up to his ribs. On the front was a huge pair of appliquéd pouty pink lips and the words "Victoria's Secret" in rhinestones. I didn't say anything because I thought that maybe *he* thought he looked jazzy. My mom saw him next, and though she did a double-take, she didn't say anything, either. I'm not sure if my dad even noticed, since he never notices what people are wearing. When we sat down to eat lunch, Isabela strolled into the kitchen and gaped at Jose.

"What are you wearing?" she shrieked. "That's my Victoria's Secret nightgown!"

Jose calmly replied, "When I get up today, it very dark, so I grab the shirt on top." He joked with Fatima that it was her fault because she was the one who had put it in his dresser drawer. He continued, "After the airport, I go to the *banco*, the *padaria* for cup *coff*, then I come home."

I giggled, but Isabela shrilled, "What? I'm so embarrassed! What are people gonna think?"

A few months later, my mom and I were in Goodwill and saw a long-sleeved red Victoria's Secret nightgown. She cut a pair of flirty lips from a piece of baby pink construction paper, taped them on the front, and mailed the nightgown to Jose, along with a note explaining that he could wear it if he had to make any winter trips to the airport. When he called, he guffawed, "I promise I gonna wear the nightgown and monkey socks on the day you move here."

In a way, humor reveals the real person. Making others laugh can make them trust you, which proved very valuable to Jose. He snatched all humor and hope from our lives. The absence of hope is a dead feeling, which is very different from feeling sad. The once-vibrant colors of my dad's world had become gray. As the "man of the family," he blamed himself for not seeing through Jose, and for getting us into this mess. He overcompensated by focusing only on making money for our family, but he didn't engage with us. He was always physically there, but he wasn't emotionally present. His spontaneity and gusto were gone. Once he started down the slippery slope of depression, it seemed hard for him to climb out of it. And I sometimes thought that he didn't want to climb back up.

Each wound—Mic's insolence and destruction, Jose's duplicity, and my grandparents' toxicity—penetrated deeper and deeper. For my mom and me, portions of our souls developed scars, but we survived. Each wound withered my dad until he contained more scar tissue than life.

In my mom and me, you couldn't really see the sadness unless you knew it was there, but that was the trick. We all had our disappointments and baggage. I wore it on my heart, my mom hid it behind a fake smile, and my dad carried it on his back.

Velya

I have always found writing to be a very cathartic experience. When we were first married and I shared pieces I had written with Jim, he would invariably comment, "It's good." That was it: "It's good." In the early years of our marriage, this used to drive me nuts. I expected him to comment on my brilliant use of metaphor, or how cleverly I had used alliteration in a certain paragraph. I now know he will always say, "It's good," just as surely as I knew he would paint our new kitchen cabinets the colonial teal I selected and loved, simply because I had selected and loved it.

As I unpacked cardboard boxes and un-bubble-wrapped pieces of our life that had been stored away for over two years, I came across a perfect example of Jim's way of offering his love to me. In our Bridgewater home, the one we had bought as newlyweds, we started a height chart to document growth on every birthday and first day of school with a ruler and black Sharpie marker. This chart had been part of the living room doorway. When we sold the house, Jim knew I could never leave this treasured memento behind, and somehow, he removed it and artfully camouflaged the spot where it had been. The height chart, a piece of our history, was now installed in the kitchen of our new house. When I walked past it and thought about what Jim had done for me, I got the same little pang I still get when he enters the room—the sensation of things flipping over a little inside my stomach.

I was a virgin when I met Jim, and have never made love with any other man. Before our lives turned upside down and we still used to laugh, we always got a kick out of the white pebble story. Long ago, I read a statistic stating that if newlyweds put a pebble *into* a bucket under their bed every time they made love that first year of marriage, and then took a pebble *out* of the bucket every time they had sex in all the remaining years of their marriage, they could never empty the bucket. "Ha!" Jim snorted. "We had the bucket empty at six months!"

We were still taking out pebbles, but I wanted to laugh like that again. I wanted the sadness to end. It covered everything, like the light film of dust that's always there on a TV screen. You can still see the picture, but things aren't clear. It was as if we each existed in a silk cocoon; yet I knew that in retreating, we were undergoing a transformation on the journey to knowing our new selves. We were both sleeping on the same *Princess and the Pea* fairytale mattress. I tried to ignore the pea of Jose's betrayal and my anger at my parents. Jim might as well have been sleeping on a boulder.

For weeks at a time, Jim barely spoke to any of us. He reminded me of the painted turtles of my childhood that sunned themselves on partially submerged logs along the shore of Rainbow Lake. He pulled his head in and withdrew from us, closing up tight for the same reasons turtles do, to protect themselves from predators. A hard shell safeguarded him now; but we would occasionally see his head poke out and catch a glimpse of the old Jim.

One night in bed, I said to his back, "You know how happy I would be if you would just say *I love you*, Jim?"

He rolled over, nuzzled my neck, and whispered in my ear, "I love you, Jim." The whole bed shook with his silent laughter and I playfully punched him in the arm.

"You're such a jerk!" I giggled. "The way you're rocking the bed reminds me of the comedian we watched that time. You laughed exactly the same way," I reminded.

"What comedian?" he asked, knowing full well what I meant. He just wanted to hear the joke again.

"The guy who said, no matter what he tried, he couldn't get rid of his girlfriend until he came up with a brilliant solution. He started peeing in her bed," I supplied.

As if hearing the lame joke for the first time, Jim shook with laughter. The whole time I talked, he circled my nipple with his tongue, and then we took a pebble out of our bucket.

But I woke to find a turtle in the bed.

We all had darkness inside of us, but, on the surface, Ehris and I were better at dealing with it than Jim. It was almost like a reverse nightmare. When you wake up from a nightmare, you're relieved. But every morning, I woke into the same crummy dream with constant mental dialogues.

If you've been up night after night with the mental torture of thoughts that go nowhere—just circling round and round in your head like a looped recording—you know that in the end, there comes a sort of quietness. You feel as if nothing, bad or good, is ever going to happen again.

CHAPTER FORTY-SIX

Ehris

"This really would have been such a nice room for Nazey," I said to my mom as we stacked unopened moving boxes in the back bedroom. "I can't believe the stupid probate judge thinks Laurel Ridge is better than this."

"Down deep, I kind of figured it would go that way, since Grandpa held her power of attorney. I can't stand coming into this room. I feel like I failed her," my mom confided.

"You didn't fail her. She never let you help her," I responded.

"She's been in Laurel Ridge for almost eighteen months now," my mom stated in a faraway voice. "She left the house with just the clothes she was wearing. She's never been back. Can you imagine leaving this house tonight and never seeing it again? And how about if you had lived here since 1960?"

I shook my head. She continued, "A tube of lipstick and Norell perfume—that's what she always had on her dresser. When we were little, she wouldn't even take a ride in the row-boat without her clip-on earrings and Cherries in the Snow lipstick. She always joked, 'You never know, Hollywood could be calling. Gregory Peck could be out there.' I remember sitting on their bed and watching her do her hair and pencil on her beauty mark. I faintly remember her using old-fashioned cake mascara that came in a red box and you had to spit on it."

"Eww, you spit on it?" I grimaced.

"Yeah, you did. But that's not the point of the story, Ehris."

"I don't get it. Like, what did you put it on with?"

"A little thing that kind of looked like a flat toothbrush," she explained.

"Wow, weird. What's so great about a nursing home?" I asked. "Nazey could be here now, with aides, living with her own family."

"I don't know, Ehris." My mom shrugged sadly.

On the day we all appeared in probate court to petition for conservatorship, Nazey wasn't there, because her court-appointed attorney said it "wasn't advisable or necessary." My mom and Uncle Jordan wanted the judge to see that although she sat in a wheelchair and drooled, Nazey knew exactly what she was saying. Uncle Jordan brought the DVD of footage they had taped the day before at Laurel Ridge, along with his laptop to play the DVD. When he asked her on camera where she wanted to live, Nazey very clearly stated, "With my daughter—with Veal and Jim." And then she told one of her favorite stories. Nazey hadn't started college until she was in her 50s, and when her British Literature professor handed back her first essay (with a grade of A+), she was so excited, she got on the exit ramp on the highway and was pulled over by a cop.

Judge Eagan, Ann Crowley-Foster, our lawyer, and the court-appointed attorney gathered around my uncle's laptop and smiled with tears in their eyes. Nazey told the story slowly, and laughed where she always did. My grandfather never rose from his seat at the conference room table. When I think of the story now, I don't see Nazey zipping past the wrong-way signs in her excitement to get home and share the news. I see my scowling grandfather with his arms crossed at the conference table, and the story is ruined for me.

Velya

My mother developed a dual personality because she married the wrong guy. When my father was around, she became guarded, and put a lid on her inquisitive side.

Our house was full of eggshells. If you've spent any time in an eggshell house, you know it's like tiptoeing through a minefield. Like a seasoned bomb-squad team leader, my mother was ever-vigilant to avoid detonating my father ("Cut the red wire. NO!! STOP!! It's not that one! Cut the blue wire!"). One minute, he could be reading The Ridgefield Press in the plaid wool wing chair. The next, he'd explode into an out-of-proportion tirade because one of the cats barfed in the kitchen, or because we kept turning on the outdoor floodlight during a snowstorm to make snow day predictions.

One sure trigger for full-blown fury was *ants*. My father was convinced that all ants were scheming carpenter ants hell-bent on eating our wavy-edge-siding house right down to its stone foundation. While my mother exalted Albert Schweitzer's reverence for life and ushered spiders outside, my father stormed around spraying Raid ("Kills 'em dead!") like it was Glade mist air freshener. I'm sure he and his fluorocarbons are partly responsible for any ozone layer holes.

One weekend morning, we were darting around in a mad rush to get out of the house as my father barked, "Let's get moving! I wanna be on the road by eight A.M.! The traffic in Hartford is gonna be brutal!" As she hurriedly opened a can of cat food, my mother noticed that she'd accidentally left the previous night's pot of pasta (sans sauce) on a back burner of the stove. The pot lid wasn't sitting properly, and when she lifted it off, she was aghast to see big black bustling ants all over the limp tangles of off-white spaghetti. Anybody who lives in the country knows that the whole animal kingdom gets going in the springtime, and the ants come marching in looking for food, warmth, and water. Every spring, my father was convinced that these ants, on coffee break from devouring our house, crawled out from their hiding places in the walls just to taunt him. So, that morning, my mother was caught between a pot full of voracious ants and my agitated ant-phobic father. One of my father's many rules (along with the rule about only using one pail of water to wash a car) forbade dumping scraps or leftovers in the woods because it would attract raccoons and skunks. My mother put the pot lid back on, scurried down to our basement, and shoved the pot in the freezer of our old extra fridge. Generally, the coating of ice around the freezer was so thick that the door wouldn't close tightly, but the week before she'd used a hair dryer and ice pick to defrost it.

A couple of weeks later (probably because she was making spaghetti again), my mother remembered the pot. The frozen-solid blob of spaghetti dotted with frozen-solid black ants was impossible to pry out, so she left it on the counter to defrost a bit. About an hour into the defrosting I heard my mom excitedly talking to herself in the kitchen, repeating, "I can't believe this! I just can't believe this!" She was hunched over the pot with her trusty jewelry loupe—the one she used to examine stuff like snowflakes, feathers, dragonfly wings, onion skins, mushroom gills, and dryer lint. "Oh my god, now what?" I muttered to myself as I joined her at the formica counter. In the aluminum pot of slush, swirls of thawing spaghetti strands wove their way between black ant corpses. Knowing she felt like a murderer, I was thinking up something comforting to say, when out of the corner of my eye, I saw an antenna wiggle. "Whoa!" I gasped. "You saw that, right?"

Pointing with a chopstick and never taking her eyes off the pot, she said, "You see that one over there? It just twitched its thorax. That other one is moving five of its legs. Somehow," she marveled, "I cryogenically preserved them!"

By the time the spaghetti was totally thawed, at least a third of the ants had totally come back to life. The process sort of reminded me of the yoga practice of savasana, the corpse pose—like waking up from a deep sleep. When you receive the inner cue to end savasana, you're supposed to gently wiggle your fingers and toes. Rock your head from side to side. Roll your body over to one side and just marinate for a few moments. Take your top hand and lift yourself up to a seated position. Sit tall, feeling happy and energetic. Be grateful for what you have just experienced, while noticing your tranquil state of mind.

Like little black Rip Van Winkles, the grateful ants waved their defrosted antennae at us. Dr. Frankenstein, aka my mom, practically had tears in her eyes. "After what they've been through, we have to set them free," she declared. We went out into the woods with the aluminum pot—and like

Joy Adamson with her beloved lioness, Elsa—my mom set the ants free on top of a rotting log. If this had been a movie, the credits would have rolled as that guy who sang "Born Free" crooned, "Born free, as free as the wind blows, as free as the grass grows, born free to follow your heart."

My father only saw the guarded version of my mother. My "real" mother emerged when he went on business trips, or when she took Jordan and me to places like the Woolworth's lunch counter where she indulged in an egg salad sandwich. The "curious" side of her was awed by the delicate lace intricacies of a spider web, and the folded front legs of a praying mantis. She even saw beauty in the thirsty two-inch long tear-drop shaped leeches that hung out in the bottom of our lake.

After decades of biting her tongue and holding back for the sake of "keeping the peace," my mother eventually lost that inquisitive side of herself. She put a permanent lid on it and just gave up.

Alone in the bedroom that would have been my mother's, I realized with total clarity that my mother had held the power, yet never used it. My father was a bully with short-man syndrome. Bullies bully in order to feel powerful, because they actually feel like nobodies. When they intimidate, threaten, or hurt someone, they feel like somebody. The key is always the feeling of power.

All my mother ever had to do was call his bluff. If, just once when he threatened her with divorce, she had said, "Fine. Pack your bags, call a lawyer, and the kids stay here with me," he would have backed right down.

Instead, my mother always made excuses for my father. His abusive father had died when he was 13, and he became the man of the family. Immediately following the funeral, in a symbolic, defiant act, he threw the cat o' nine tails his father used to beat him with into the coal stove. Yet until he joined the Marine Corps at the start of World War II, he terrorized his younger brother and berated his mother. He was never held accountable for his actions, and my mother always said we should feel sorry for him.

Then I had a darker thought. What if, all along, my mother *knew* she held the power, but chose not to use it? What if she felt she deserved to be punished in her marriage? *Mothers love their children—they don't abandon them.* She must have done something *very bad* in order to drive her own mother away. She must have felt she deserved to be treated badly by her husband in order to atone.

And then, an even darker thought—*but what about us?*

CHAPTER FORTY-SEVEN

Velya

❀

Ehris is one of those effortlessly beautiful young women—the kind who can wear yoga pants and have it be a fashion choice, not a sloppy one. She settled herself on the couch next to me, folding her legs under her. Her makeup-free face was flushed from a shower, and she tucked a damp wayward curl behind her ear. She knew I could tell with one glance, one look. It was her eyes. They were dark-rimmed, haunted, and sad.

"I feel like you and I are alone in the world," she said, sniffling and beginning to cry. "Everybody else has gone crazy. How could any of this have happened?"

"I don't know, Ehris," I admitted. "But think about all the wonderful people out there, too. What about Guilherme? He was a total stranger, but he helped us in the long run."

"Yeah, that's true," Ehris agreed. "He did finally sell the farm and sent us some of the money."

"Think about the huge thank-you party we're having for all the people who've helped us since we've been back. I'm starting to think that what Uncle Jordan said is true. Daddy and I wish you *could* have been spared all the heartache, but at the same time, you've been given an early lesson in the realities of life, and maybe that's not so bad. The beautiful things and the kindness of others become more special when you know how dark the flip side can be."

"I can't believe you're wiping snot off my face with your *hands*," she spluttered.

"Maybe it's because I love you that much," I whispered into her hair.

Curled up like an elegant cat, Ehris was pretty, but pretty alone is not what people saw in her. It might seem like an inappropriate thing for a mother to say about her own daughter, but she was seductive, and her seduction stemmed from the fact that she was totally unaware of her iridescence.

"Ehris, you'll never allow yourself to become the invisible, silent woman that Nazey was, because you love and value yourself. I want you to keep humming with dreams and ideas like you always have."

Because we were fluent in each other's language, I didn't take offense when she said, "I feel like there's no one else to talk to except you. Everyone else has gotten so weird!"

Ehris

The more a daughter knows about her mother's life, the stronger the daughter. For me, the time before my mom became my mom is a string of stories, told and retold: the time she accidentally kidnapped a "lost" basset hound from its own yard; the time she added too much yeast to the root beer brewing in the basement, and the bottles exploded all over the ceiling; the night she and her friends were driving

around in a cemetery, somehow impaled the car on a headstone, then dug up the headstone to dislodge the car (and
that week's *Ridgefield Press* reported the disturbed grave as
"cemetery vandalism"). The old photos of her, even the one
with the shag haircut and red flowered maxi skirt she was
forced to make in Home Ec, stood as an historical record of
the person she was before me. These photos accompany the
legends. Because any story about your mom is part legend,
isn't it?

I once heard that the way mothers speak to their daughters becomes their inner voice, and that's certainly true for
me. Whenever I'm thinking about trying something new, it's
my mom's voice I hear pointing out the endless possibilities, assuring me that I can do it, that I have the power, and
reminding me that failing is not nearly as bad as never making an attempt. "There's no growth without change, Ehris,"
I can hear her say. The worst thing in life must be to have a
mother who discourages you, instills fear in you, holds you
back, pushes you down, and never encourages you to fly.

CHAPTER FORTY-EIGHT

Velya

❖

Normally, I visited Laurel Ridge late at night, because that was when my mother hated it the most. Most times, I'd show up around 10:00 P.M. Stuffy air smelling of bleach and meatloaf always hit me as I walked through the sliding doors. As nursing homes go, Laurel Ridge was probably a decent place, but nothing said *the 1980s* faster than the riot of mauve roses that bombarded visitors upon entering the lobby. A six-inch-wide Laura Ashley wallpaper border in shades of sea foam, teal, peach, and coral hung at the ceiling in a pattern that carried over to the fabrics on the puffy balloon valances and roll-arm love seats. It was suffocating.

It wasn't any better once you got past the lobby. I usually wheeled my mother to a room decorated in burgundy, hunter green, and navy. Geese in gingham scarves adorned the throw pillows. The Harlequin romance and Danielle Steel paperbacks on the glossy polyurethaned bookshelf never appeared to circulate.

When I showed up late at night, I was able to bypass the unstaffed reception desk, ignore the sign-in book, enter the keypad access code to the dementia ward, and spend time with my mother at a much quieter point in the day. There was no blaring overhead paging system. I didn't have to hear a patient ask for a bedpan, or an overworked, underpaid aide respond that she was busy, so "Just pee in the diaper, because that's what it's there for." The chipper woman who strummed "Row, Row, Row Your Boat" on her acoustic guitar to a roomful of adults had gone home.

I'm sure you've heard the old joke. What do nursing homes smell like? Depends. I didn't have a problem with Laurel Ridge. It wasn't *their* fault my mother was there and not at home where she could have been—where she was supposed to be. They appeared to take decent care of their patients, but it was a transitional place between life and death. There was an all-encompassing feeling, once you passed the sliding doors, that death was coming and no one cared. At night, when the world was gray, it seemed a fitting time at Laurel Ridge for someone to slip free, to just let go. I didn't see it as a bad thing.

Today, I was at Laurel Ridge in the morning. My mother sat so small in her wheelchair, hands clasped in her lap. I bent to kiss her, and saw shining scalp between sparse wisps of hair. I remembered the pin curls she bobby-pinned to her scalp every night. Her breasts, which had once stood so firm and proud, were now empty sacks. Her boobs had been pretty incredible, and Jordan recently told me that boys on our school bus called our mother "Torpedo Tits." That still makes me smile.

Dueling TV channels blared in the room my mother shared with a stranger. $12,000 a month bought a "semi-private" space that looked like a hospital room with the beds separated by a piece of fabric.

I wheeled my mother to the burgundy room, where we sat side-by-side as she held my hand and slowly twirled my wedding ring around my finger. She looked up at me with squinted eyes and asked, "You're still married?"

"Of course I am, Mom. I'll always be married to Jim."

"That's not what Daddy told me," she said haltingly, as I helped her wipe drool from the side of her mouth. Her drooling embarrassed my father, and he constantly leapt from his seat to dab it away.

I said very slowly, "I don't think you should believe all the things Daddy tells you."

Her eyes fixed on the drool cloth in her lap. I wheeled her chair directly in front of me so we could sit face-to-face. I bent down low and held her hands. She tilted her head a bit and in a tiny voice pleaded, "When am I going home?"

The truth was hanging in the air. Maybe it wasn't my secret to tell. But maybe it was, because my parents' secrets had made secrets in my life, too. Maybe they weren't secrets, but silences—and how is that any different than a lie?

"I think the time for lies and secrets is over, Mom. Someone has to tell you the truth. Daddy will never bring you home. We lost our case in probate court because he holds your power of attorney. I can't get you out of here until Daddy dies. You're not going home."

I knew she wouldn't be emotional. She always took great pride in her Scottish heritage, and boasted that the women in her family were strong and never cried.

"I want you to go to the house," she said with surprising strength.

"No, I don't want to see Daddy."

"He won't be there. He's getting a new bumper on the car."

"Why do you want me to go to the house?"

"I want the copy of *Black Beauty* from Babe. It's on the bookshelf in your room. Get it for me."

"Oh, yeah, the one she gave you when you were little. Remember how that was the first chapter book I read? I loved that story. It always cracked me up how she signed it 'Aunt Babe,' even though she was only four years older than you."

My mother nodded and turned her head away.

"Okay, okay, I'll get it for you. I'll bring it with me next time I come."

"Go now," she commanded. "Get it today."

She closed her eyes, and I knew our conversation was over.

I had never taken the key to my parents' house off my keychain, even though I hadn't been there since my mother had been shipped off to Laurel Ridge. For just a moment, I took comfort in the familiarity of the house's smell. There are things you can't forget that you wish you could. The broken pieces of the amber long-stemmed cocktail glass were still inside of me. I looked at the dining room floor where it had shattered, and every time I took a breath, they stabbed into me. *Get the book and get out of here*, I told myself.

The banister still creaked at the exact same place. Anxious to get out of the house before my father returned, I thought, *Ha! I wonder what he did to the car this time?* Several years before, he had been impatient for a flock of Canada geese to cross the road. Rather than just wait, he tried to pass them, and scraped the entire length of the car's passenger side on a concrete bridge. He was always doing stupid, impulsive stuff like that without thinking about the consequences. Committing my mother to Laurel Ridge and thinking all would be hunky-dory within the family was the finest example of his impetuousness.

My room looked exactly the same, right down to the pink and yellow flower-power wallpaper I had picked out when I was 11. Nothing had changed on my bookshelf. My fingers touched my favorites: *Wuthering Heights, The Grapes of Wrath, A Tree Grows in Brooklyn,* and then the cloth-covered edition of *Black Beauty.* Pulling it from the shelf, I knew exactly what was inscribed on the inside cover.

September 19, 1936
Happy Birthday, Neysa!
With love,
Your "Aunt" Babe

August 23, 1964
For Veal,
On her first reading birthday...
Love,
Mommy

Aunt Babe had given the book to my mother on her tenth birthday, and my mother had passed it on to me when I turned six. We had very few family heirlooms, and this book had always been important to me. I had felt very grown up when I first read it and was introduced to Black Beauty, Ginger, Squire Gordon, and young Joe Green.

Holding the book, I sat on my twin bed and knew that home, as I had known it, was gone. Home is a place where you feel at peace, but if you go back there after the people are gone, then all you can see is what's not there anymore, and maybe never was. There were eggshells scattered all over my rug, and they had been on the stairs as I made my way to my room. For the first time in this house, I hadn't avoided them. I'd crushed them beneath my feet. The crunching was exhilarating! Home is a place where you want to be, and I did not want to be there.

I noticed a bookmark in *Black Beauty*, and opened to the page. A stamped white legal envelope addressed to me at our old Bridgewater address, and written in my father's hand, slipped from the book. *What the heck is this?* I wondered. Curious, I opened the envelope that had already been unsealed, unfolded a piece of white-lined paper, and read:

Velya,

No grandson of mine is a goddamn fag! How can I hold my head up around my friends if I have to watch him prance around on stage like that? Your son is dead to me and you failed as his mother.

Your father

The flower-power wallpaper spun around me, yet time stopped. I read the note again as *Black Beauty* slipped to the floor. In the stillness of my bedroom, my mother's voice came to me: "I can handle Daddy." I knew exactly what had happened, because I knew my mother. She had surreptitiously taken the letter out of the mailbox after my father had left for the gym and before the mailman picked it up — that was why there was no postmark.

Hold his head up around his friends? What friends? My father literally did not have a single friend. But then, why would I be surprised? Everything had always been about him and his inadequacies with himself.

It was so clear to me now. Mic had been involved in all of the theater productions in high school, and there came a time when my father just stopped going. None of us really gave it too much thought, because he would rarely go and see Jordan perform, either—that is, unless Jordan was able to comp tickets for him.

I thought of the birthday and Christmas money for Mic that my mother would press into my hand, always in the pantry or their bathroom, always in ten-dollar bills, whispering, "Tell Mic not to worry anymore about writing thank-you notes. We remember how busy this time of life is for young people."

Once she entered Laurel Ridge, all communication with both Ehris and Mic had stopped. I had just chalked it up to my father never having been the one to take care of those things.

Rising from the bed, I walked to the window to look at the lake. My life had revolved around the lake and this room for all of my growing-up years. I had left my baby teeth under the pillow in this room. I had put on my wedding dress in this room...but this was a house, not a home. It's not home if you want to run away from it.

I was surprisingly calm when I picked up *Black Beauty* from the floor.

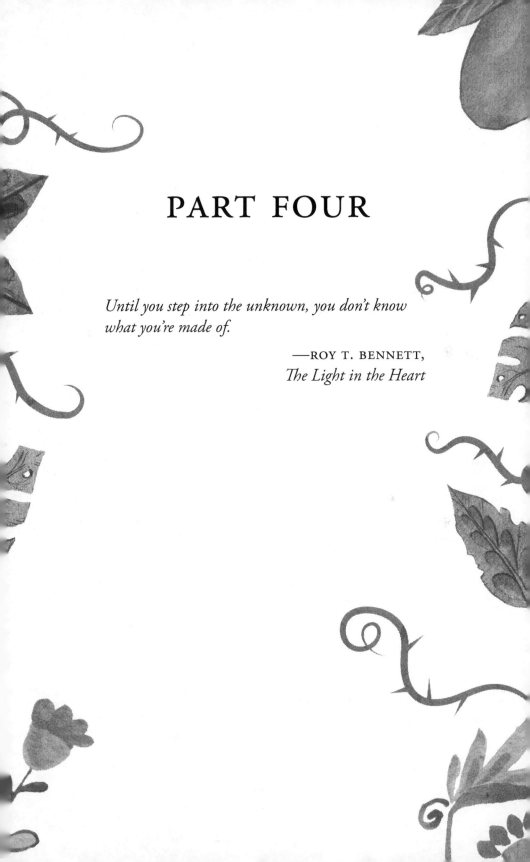

PART FOUR

Until you step into the unknown, you don't know
what you're made of.

—ROY T. BENNETT,
The Light in the Heart

CHAPTER FORTY-NINE

Velya

An orderly was carrying what looked to be an untouched lunch tray from my mother's room when I blew in. As usual, my parents weren't speaking to each other. My mother was zoned out in her wheelchair, and my father was glaring at Fox News from across the room.

Crossing the room and throwing the envelope at my father's feet I said, "My gay son is a finer man than you will ever be. You talk about holding your head up?! You're a pathetic excuse for a human being!" Turning to my mother, who was instantly coherent, I said, "Lies and secrets, Mom, they're like gangrene. They eat away what is good, and leave only destruction behind. Sometimes, you have to amputate the foot to save the leg. I have to amputate you in order to save Jim, Ehris, Mic, and myself. I can't do this anymore and I think you know that, and it's why you had me find the letter. You knew it was the final straw. No decent mother would allow her child to be attacked that way. I know you didn't write the letter, you just took it out of the mailbox. But it's not enough, Mom. You never took a stand. You were either so in love with Daddy, or so afraid he'd leave you, that you didn't care what happened to us. Every moment of our lives we make choices. Some of your choices are beyond explanation—like choosing your husband over your kids."

I bent and kissed her on the cheek. Then, looking into her eyes I said, "Mom, I have to become whole again. The secrets in your life have eaten you alive, and I won't let that happen to me, or to my family. Remember your index cards? Your 'walk away from destructive people' index cards? I'm doing that, Mom. I'm walking away and I can't come back."

I rose, looked at them both for the last time, then left the room. Before I got to the mauve lobby, I had already cut the decaying gangrenous tissue from my life, and was left with a raw stump. *Maybe, like a starfish, I'll grow a new leg*, I thought as the sliding doors opened for the final time. And then, I threw up in the parking lot of Laurel Ridge.

CHAPTER FORTY-SEVEN

Velya

❁

Outside of family, I was always reluctant to discuss three significant topics in my life: alternative medicine, atheism, and Mic's homosexuality. I was hesitant to talk about these subjects because when I did, other people got all squirmy and uneasy. I felt bad about making them uncomfortable. Kind of dopey, huh? *I* felt bad about making *them* uncomfortable.

For years, my family politely listened to Christian songs performed at public school winter concerts. At secular school graduations, I sat quietly during benedictions. I simply omitted the words "under God" whenever I said the "Pledge of Allegiance," and never complained about Congress changing its original wording to include "one nation under God" in 1954. An enlightening acupuncture session made me decide to finally stop worrying about other people's uneasiness.

My new acupuncturist, Andrea, needled me—in a good way. At private acupuncture sessions, I had always felt like a patient—a person who was sick, but she offered community acupuncture, and I knew it was the place for me as soon as I walked in the door. Like snoozing porcupines, five clients at a time lounged in recliners draped with sage-colored sheets. This community acupuncture approach was more like driving in to Jiffy Lube for a quick oil change and a little preventative maintenance.

Andrea was trying to help me deal with my grief and balance my *chi*, or circulating life energy. Everything was fine during the day. It was only at night, when the house was still, that my brain wandered over to the danger zone.

After my first appointment, I felt tremendous relief. It's hard to explain, but it was as if a forcefield had been created in my head. It was like I was in a *Star Trek* episode with Captain Kirk at the helm of the USS Enterprise—nothing could get through. All negative thoughts bounced off the forcefield, even when they tried to conceal themselves in cloaking devices.

At my next appointment, Andrea inserted needles in various parts of my body and said seriously, "We have to keep your organs balanced. We don't want you dried out. We want to keep you moist and buoyant."

"Moist and buoyant," I tittered.

At that moment, she inserted a needle at the base of my bottom left rib, the liver chi.

"Whoa!" she observed, and I felt an intense itchiness at the point where the needle had gone in. "I wish you could see this! You have a mark the size and shape of a croissant, with the exact redness and shininess of a third-degree burn. This is good!"

"It is?" I asked.

"Yes, something toxic is working its way free." She explained that anger and repressed frustrations cause the liver chi to stagnate, and that when we are in perfect health, all the chi energy runs harmoniously throughout the body.

I spent the next 60 minutes in a recliner in a very relaxed state, thinking about what I was repressing and dying to see the elusive red mark. I caught myself quietly snoring, and then, out of the blue, a table conversation at a recent wedding popped into my mind. I don't follow any sports or teams, but since we live in Connecticut, a major topic of conversation is college basketball. I responded to the guy seated next to me, "The only sport Jim faithfully watches is UConn women's basketball, primarily because he likes Geno Auriemma's coaching style."

"Women's basketball? What's wrong with him? Is he gay, or something?" my tablemate sneered.

It's not necessary to point out the stupidity of this comment, let alone the inappropriateness. However, I knew how embarrassed this guy's wife would have been if I had called him on it, so I just ignored the comment. I ignored the sexist, offensive comment so other people at the wedding, a joyous celebration, would not be uncomfortable. All weekend, I thought about this. I had let this guy get away with something that was wrong on so many levels. He had insulted women's sports teams, Jim, and our gay kid. I didn't speak up and hold this man accountable. I contributed to a culture of silence that says it's not okay to make waves or swim against the tide.

We often choose silence because we dread awkward conversations. We fear them, because experience has taught us that if we open up and are honest, bad things may happen. So we choose silence.

As I stared at the ceiling and thought about the flaming red croissant on my left side, I realized bad things were happening inside of *me*, and that was the risk of not speaking up.

The New Age music without corners or sharp edges and the soothing warmth of the clinic helped me drift away into a contemplative state. The *first they came* quotation attributed to Pastor Martin Niemoller entered my thoughts:

> *"First they came for the communists,*
> *and I didn't speak out because I wasn't a communist.*
>
> *Then they came for the trade unionists,*
> *and I didn't speak out because I wasn't a trade unionist.*
>
> *Then they came for the Jews,*
> *and I didn't speak out because I wasn't a Jew.*
>
> *Then they came for me,*
> *and there was no one left to speak out for me."*

I signaled that I was ready, and Andrea removed my needles. I had that euphoric post-acupuncture feeling as I drove home, and realized that it's okay for people to feel uncomfortable. Examining one's thoughts and feelings can be extremely unsettling, and so can honest conversation, but those uncomfortable moments force us to think and grow. Aristotle wrote, "It is the mark of an educated mind to be able to entertain a thought without accepting it." I never expected anyone to accept my beliefs, but just as my family sat politely through those Christian songs year after year, I expected courtesy in return. The person I had become could not remain silent. I knew, firsthand, what keeping the peace and not rocking the boat could do to a woman. That woman would never be me.

CHAPTER FIFTY-ONE

Velya

❀

"Hey," Mic said when he called, "can someone pick me up at LaGuardia on Tuesday at 5:30? I can't wait to see you guys! I can't wait to see the house!"

"Of course one of us will pick you up, and we can't wait to see you, either," I said. "If I'm not home when you get here, you have to swear not to go in the house without me. I'm dying to see your first reaction."

"Mommy," he laughed. "I swear I will wait in the driveway until you come home."

"You promise?"

"I swear on Norma's head," Mic chuckled, invoking a solemn oath he, Ehris, and I had invented years ago. Norma had been a favorite cat, and somehow this had become an honorary pledge we never broke. It was our version of swearing on the Bible.

"Okay, that's good enough for me. You want steak on the grill, and apple crisp for dessert, right?" I asked, already knowing the answer.

"*Your* apple crisp," he corrected. "Nobody makes it like you."

"Oh, brother, you just want me to double the recipe." I smiled into the phone.

"Of course, and hey Mommy, don't do any decorating without me, okay?"

"Mic, it's a twelve-room house! Believe me, we'll be decorating for a long time to come. We love you. See you Tuesday," I said, and hung up.

Mic had always been my larger-than-life flamboyant child. He actually once asked if he could get Botox injections in his armpits to cure his allegedly terrible sweatiness that I had never noticed. Of course, he made this cockamamie request as I was cooking dinner with a Great Dane puppy and a hungry cat underfoot, while simultaneously helping Ehris glue dried parsley to the bottom of a shoebox to simulate the African grasslands for some diorama she was making. He was offended I didn't take him seriously.

Jim was working late, so at the airport, I helped Mic load his suitcase and backpack into the trunk of our car, staggering under their weight. "Let me guess what's in there—fifty pounds of forks?"

"And the hammer, pliers, and vice," he laughed. "Yo, you can't believe the amazing ones I got at this junky antique store in Old San Juan. I found a lot of those patterns I love like Persia, Siren, Lakewood, and La Vigne."

Mic owned his own business called *Silverwear Antique Fork Jewelry*. He made up-cycled jewelry, primarily fork bracelets, from vintage silver-plate flatware. He began by selling at the University of Puerto Rico. As word spread, he was invited to sell in boutiques and shops all over Puerto Rico, and then expanded to the New England area. My unique neoclassical Venus fork bracelet, which I always wore, had generated many sales.

Mic loved the entire process, and spent happy weekend mornings scouring flea markets, haggling with vendors, and then proudly displaying his loot for us to see when he got home. He loved creating the bracelets as well as the photography and marketing, and had established a very profitable niche market for himself. Someone had given him *The Book of Silver Flatware Silver Marks & Patterns*, which listed the names and dates of virtually all silverware patterns. He pored over it in the same way Wolfgang Puck probably gobbled up cookbooks. I had once heard him tell a flea market vendor, "Excuse me, but did you know that soup ladle is the Saint Cloud pattern by Gorham from 1874, and it's worth $219? It's sterling, not plate, and you really shouldn't let it go for the price you have on the tag."

From the passenger seat, he chattered, "As soon as we get home, we should get rid of all the stainless steel silverware and use nothing but mismatched silver plate. How cool would that be? I'll give you all the pieces I have that are too hard to bend, and we can keep adding to them. We really should be using vintage silverware, don't ya think, since it's my business? Hey, did you hear I said *home*? That word sounds pretty nice, doesn't it?"

"It certainly does," I answered, pulling onto the highway, which was busy with rush hour traffic. "Hey Mic, quick... look behind you...can I change lanes?"

"Yeah, relax. Pull over after that green Subaru. Oh man, remember the time we drove to Hartford and you were freaking out and your knuckles were white and you made me feel the sweat on your forehead?" he sassed.

"Like I always tell you guys—*you* learned to drive from calm Daddy. *I* learned to drive from neurotic Grandpa. And yes, I'll be very happy with us all under one roof."

He laughed, "Dude, you know, in all three years, nobody in the dorm floor above or below me ever asked about all the pounding that went on in my room when I hammered the forks."

"I'm not your dude," I corrected. "But nobody complained? That's pretty weird!"

"You'd love my friend Rosario. She's so cool. She's working on her master's, and she's a stripper at night," he disclosed.

"Is she any good? Did you see her?"

"She's six feet tall, so I bet she looked pretty good on a stripper pole. We were all going to check out her show, but she wanted to perfect her act first, and then I left to come home."

"Wouldn't it be kind of creepy to watch a friend strip?" I asked, glancing in the rearview mirror.

"She just got two Chihuahua puppies and gave them both the same name," he reported. I digested this, and thought she sounded a lot like George Foreman, whose five sons were all named George. This was the thing about Mic—you would start a conversation with him and it could go in 15 directions, but I could always keep up, since I was the same way.

"She was great. I could always count on her. Like one time, I had to make a last-minute delivery to one of my boutiques, and I was like, 'Yo, Rosario. I'm in a jam and need a ride to the rainforest,' and she came and picked me up."

"Mic," I laughed, shaking my head, "who says that kind of stuff?"

"What kind of stuff?" he asked.

"Who says, 'Yo, I need a ride to the rainforest?'"

My colorful child was home.

The four of us made up for lost time and entertained often. The old house was alive with guests, and Jim was never quite sure who he'd find at the dinner table when he came home from work. Ehris and I whipped up favorite family recipes and giggled at notations in the margins of our cookbooks: *Jim devoured; almost good but a bit too molassesy; Ehris's second favorite dessert; good way to use up bananas; jazz it up; moist and easy; makes two loaves; everyone loved it!; G-r-e-a-t! Yummy!; Very good with chopped broccoli, too!; Ha!—good luck getting this one out of the pan!*

Our company always seemed reluctant to leave, and stayed later than they intended. It was as if the house embraced them and held them close. Everyone asked the same question when we gave them the tour: "Why in the world was this house empty for five years?"

Sometimes Ehris and Mic cooked midnight feasts for their friends, and I cursed them as I wiped up splattered olive oil or found an inch of milk left in the half-gallon jug. One morning, just as I was about to flit downstairs in my underwear to let our hungry cats in the house, I caught a glimpse of a guy sleeping in the guest room. Milk had disappeared, friends had appeared, and lights were on everywhere. These were the telltale signs of teenagers in the house—floors strewn with dirty clothes, plus all the drama, mess, and stray people their lives embodied.

They scattered, like cats at a dog show, sensing an impending explosion as I muttered and cleaned up yet another kitchen mess *I* hadn't made. Then I stopped, the purple sponge still warm in my hand from its rinse under the faucet. I remembered one of my mother's index cards that used to hang on the refrigerator in their home. She had used her Royal typewriter to copy a quotation that popped into my mind:

Most delightful things are messy: children, dogs, woods, and mulberry trees. Hospitals and graveyards are neat.

~KATHERINE DUNFORD

What was I getting so worked up about? The olive oil had splattered when Mic was cooking mushroom and broccoli omelets for his friends. It wasn't like they were having Twinkies and beer for breakfast! Both kids had full-time jobs and were incredible people.

Hospitals and graveyards are neat....

These were the final years of cherished family dinners with darting conversations only the four of us could follow. Our nightly exchanges reminded me of the flickering fireflies dancing just past the patio table as we floated through the years and remembered, reminisced, recalled. All it took was a mentioned memory, and we were off to another topic as the glow of the previous topic extinguished without dying. These were intimate dinners with loved ones—so private they were practically clandestine.

These days were slipping through my fingers, and I was worried about the stupid electric bill and mounds of clothes on bedroom floors. Had all we'd been through taught me nothing? Precious time was going by and one day, too soon, the house would be tidy. Jim and I didn't splatter olive oil, but neither did we burst, blaze, and glow with goals and dreams.

After Mic had been home for about a month, I came home to a kitchen that was a mess once again. Cocoa powder dusted the backsplash and blobs of batter formed cryptic

Rorschach inkblots on the marble counter. As I watched from the living room, a glorious pair of tanned legs glided from the pantry to the oven to the dishwasher. I remembered those legs when they were little and chubby, dotted with mosquito bites and crusty scabs. Ehris had offered to make cupcakes for dessert. Part of me wanted to leap from the couch and wipe something up, and the other part knew that before too long, those glorious legs wouldn't be in my kitchen, and I didn't want to wipe away any of the memories.

CHAPTER FIFTY-TWO

Velya

Paying the property tax bill in person at Woodbury Town Hall started me on my compulsive path to researching our home. It was mid-August, and I had put off writing the huge check as long as possible. As I handed my paperwork to the woman in the tax collector's office, I casually asked if she knew how to go about researching the house we had just purchased. It turned out that the woman was a member of the town's historical society.

"Follow me to the vault in the town clerk's office," she beckoned. "That's where all the land deeds are stored."

A *vault?!* My imagination got the best of me, and I was expecting to be taken to some cool brick-lined underground room with an arched stone ceiling and heavy iron gates. In reality, it was just a room filled with bound ledgers, bright fluorescent ceiling lights, and slanted wooden architect-type drafting tables. I guess I was thinking of a crypt, not a vault.

When I told the woman the address of our house, she flipped through a three-ring binder organized by street names. My eyes widened when she showed me that a preliminary investigation had been completed on our house in order to include it in the National Register of Historic Places.

She turned the page, handing me the binder. The *Solomon Minor house c. 1770*?! Holy guacamole! That's where we *live*! The typed report said it was a *three-bay, ridge-to-street Colonial-style home built about 1770. This house has historical and architectural significance as one of the oldest houses in Woodbury.* I felt giddy as I jumped ahead to read, *It was built about 1770 for Solomon Minor at the time of his marriage to Mary Root. His father deeded him this lot in 1773, which already included Solomon's house.*

"Take your time in here. I'll make a copy of the report for you," the woman said as she walked out of the vault.

Why hadn't the realtor included this information in the property listing? We actually lived in a house built before the American Revolution! The car practically drove itself home as I kept glancing at the photocopy on the passenger seat. As luck would have it, nobody was home when I got there, and I was bursting with excitement. My mind wandered as I started making a salad and setting the table for dinner.

The house took on an entirely different feel as I looked around the kitchen. Ice damage from the previous winter had been a blessing in disguise. The kitchen ceiling had gotten wet and Jim had had to pull down the soggy sheetrock. When he did, he had discovered the ceiling's original hand-hewn log beams. It was a messy job, but the beams became the focal point of the kitchen, and we loved them. I was in awe of the logs that still had strips of bark on them. I marveled at the thought that Mary Root Minor had probably seen the beams installed, and may even have touched the bark. Perhaps her husband, Solomon, had actually chopped down the trees. Suspended from square-cut nails we had found hammered into the timbers were bundles of herbs from Ehris's garden. I trailed my hand along them. Waves of anise hyssop, fennel, and lavender filled the air. Now, alone in the kitchen with the town hall paperwork in hand, I could almost see the feather frost on the windowpanes and braids of onions drying on rafters as a side of venison aged in the chimney smoke. It was such a feeling of connection and validation. I was officially hooked.

"Can you imagine the conversations that went on here?" Mic asked after hearing about the town hall discovery.

"They probably talked about the Boston Tea Party, the Stamp Act, the Declaration of Independence, all that stuff," Ehris agreed as she passed the salad bowl.

"I was thinking that, too," I said, "and then I started thinking about the Civil War, the Great Depression, when Pearl Harbor was bombed...."

Mic jumped in. "That's right! People lived through all of that in this house."

"And even the stuff that's not historical, like all the New Year's Eves, breakfasts, and birthday cakes that happened here," said Ehris.

"There must have been barns out there somewhere, too. I wonder how much land the property originally had," Jim said with an enthusiasm I hadn't seen in over two years.

"Well, here's my plan," I explained. "The lady at town hall said there's all kinds of information at the library, and I may be able to trace the property back to the original deed at the town clerk's office."

"Yo, you guys! How amazing would it be to find the deed from 1770?" Mic said excitedly.

"I know, I was thinking that while I was driving home. Isn't this like so cool?"

"I don't understand why they didn't include this stuff in the listing," Jim mused. "If buyers had known the house was built in 1770 and research has been started on it, maybe the bank wouldn't have had to keep lowering and lowering the price."

Of course, I was waiting at the town clerk's office when they unlocked the doors the next morning. An affable woman gave me a crash course on how to trace all the previous owners of our house. By researching the most recent deed for the property, I could search for the current name of the person holding the title: the grantee. Then, I could search for the grantor's name in the grantee's book to find when the title had transferred ownership. This all sounded very complicated, but once I got the hang of it, it was just working backward through time. I should have packed a lunch.

Before too long, I had taken over three of the long tables with open ledgers, and began filling out the form to request pages I wanted the town clerk to photocopy. I felt like an archaeologist, peeling back layers and uncovering names from the past. In 1958, our house had sold for $25,000 and included 35.4 acres. In 1898, it had included 45 acres and sold for "a valuable sum." In 1883, a "promissory note of $875.00 payable on demand with interest annually at five percent" was placed on the house. I found handwritten dog licenses dating from 1850 to 1880. *Dog licenses existed during the Civil War?!* Brown and white hunting dogs named Jack, Prince, and Duke had once lived at our house. I learned the names and descriptions of the dogs, but sadly, not their mistresses. The first deeds I found were typed, but the ones prior to 1919, written by hand in old-fashioned loopy cursive, became intrinsically personal. I could almost see personality in their ornamental penmanship.

In 1854, eight different heirs had signed the deed and witnessed the transfer of property, and in 1821, Solomon Minor had deeded the property to his son but reserved "life-use to myself and my second wife, Olive, as long as she remains my widow." I thought about all the events that had transpired in that 1958 to 1821 period. From Elvis Presley's induction in the army to the swearing-in of James Monroe for the second term of his presidency, I had gone back through time.

It took an entire day, but finally I reached the end—in reality, the beginning—of my quest. I found the final brown leather ledger I was hunting for, and pulled it from a metal shelf. I held my breath as I opened Volume 18 and carefully, almost reverently, turned to page 216. *Holy mackerel!* It was there! The deed was very hard to read, for sprinkled (or *fprinkled*) throughout was the letter *f* in words like *finged*, *fealed*, and *faid*, or signed, sealed, and said. From a college linguistics class, I remembered this *f* was actually called a "long s" and dated back to the Middle Ages. I could almost picture the goose quill ink pen a man named Gideon Small had used to record the transaction.

Solomon Minor was deeded land, which included a house and garden, from his father, Matthew Minor, on February 16, 1773 for the consideration of "love, goodwill, and parental affection which I have and do have unto my loving son Solomon Minor of said Woodbury, Connecticut" in the "colony of Connecticut in the 13th year of the reign of our Sovereign Lord George the Third of Great Britain." Solomon's land totaled 85 acres and 35 rods, and bordered the highway, a brook, David Turner's pasture, and a white oak. *Colony of Connecticut? King George the Third?* I couldn't believe I had done it!

That night after dinner, we excitedly studied the photocopies of all the deeds, and did our best to decipher them. Even with a magnifying glass, there were words we couldn't make out due to the handwriting and unfamiliar terms, but it didn't matter; we were elated, and anxious to learn more.

"Eighty-five acres," Jim pondered. "The land must have gone across the road, down to the river, and way back behind the house."

"Yo, Ehris!" said Mic. "Remember how every single year in school we studied the American Revolution?"

"Yeah!" Ehris answered. "I never thought King George the Third would actually appear in our lives!"

"I think I'm still kind of in shock," I said. "It's a weird feeling to sort of spend all that time in the past and then come back to the present. I'm definitely going to the library tomorrow to see if I can find out anything about Mary Root Minor and her family. At the town hall, they said that's where all those kinds of records are kept."

What I hadn't explained to my family was that the history of our house was beginning to consume me. I wasn't losing my marbles, but Jim adamantly refused to talk about Jose or my parents. The research was a form of self-therapy. I time-traveled so far back that I lost myself in other people's lives.

CHAPTER FIFTY-THREE

Velya

At the end of August, Hurricane Irene made her destructive way up the east coast. Except for the firehouse, where residents were able to take showers, our little town of Woodbury was completely shut down for four days.

As I entered the steamy concrete firehouse bathroom for my hurried shower on day three of no power, I noticed an artfully arranged basket of assorted shampoos, bath gels, and lotions outside the shower stall. Such a small gesture, yet a much-needed oasis of prettiness during a week of darkness. Women are good at that. The next night, there was a bowl of tampons, a purple blow dryer, and some gourmet chocolates. That basket of feminine goodies, and the woman who put it there, stayed with me all week.

Each night as I sat in our dark house, I thought about the women who had come before me. They didn't get a tingle of relief when the power finally came back on. There was no gleeful flushing of toilets or a leisurely hot shower. They dealt with the exhausting repetition of daily life, every day. Having grown up in Connecticut, I had lost power many times before, but losing power in this house was different.

We had given our generator to a family in Brazil who had befriended us. Cars weren't driving by, the refrigerator wasn't humming, nothing came out of the faucet, and there were no phone calls or internet. There was no gas, and all the restaurants were closed. Squinting to read by candlelight got old pretty quickly. With the hand-hewn log beams above and the wide-board floors below, it was almost possible to get a tiny taste of what life must have been like in colonial days. The past is closer in an old house.

The week before the hurricane, Jim accepted a job as operations manager for a fencing company and had to run an entire facility that, for seven days, wound up being without lights, computers, or phones. The town library got their power back days before we did, so I started hanging out there. I could go to the bathroom, actually flush the toilet, and even drink from the water fountain! In my search for colonial history, I discovered a riveting book published in 1899 called *Home Life in Colonial Days* by Alice Morse Earle. The last time the book had been checked out was in 1964. It had that musty, inky smell of an old book. I knew it would be good just from the smell of it. Woodbury Library had all kinds of out-of-the-way little places to lose yourself in a good book, and I did just that.

I also came across a little black book published in 1898 called *Barnes' Mortality Record of the Town of Woodbury, From the Settlement of the Town of Woodbury in 1672, to the Present Day.* This little book was one of the most heartbreaking yet fascinating accounts of colonial life I had ever seen. It was simply a chronological list of deaths in the town of Woodbury, but it revealed so much more. I became witness to the grim reality of life in the colonies with the very first entry, which listed the death of a baby girl followed by the death of her mother eight days later.

August 19, 1678 Esther, daughter of Samuel Galpin
August 27, 1678 Esther, wife of Samuel Galpin

As I read on, I thought, *life is difficult for women today, but at least we all have first names!*

April 18, 1780 Benjamin Judson's wife
March 9, 1781 Israel Martin's wife
October 16, 1783 Widow Hurd
February 23, 1788 Child of Richard Peet

Speaking of names, there were the predictable ones we've come to associate with that era: Mary, Hannah, Margaret, Sarah, and Martha. But oh, what a rich assortment of unusual names I uncovered: Experience, Hepzibah, Thankful, Submit, Mercy, Jemima, Jerusha, Patience, Clarinda, Birdesy, Lulu Belle, Lottie, Thirza, Dothy, Mehetabel, Betterus, Preserved Strong, and Currence.

Most of the entries simply listed dates, names, and age at death, but the cause of death was included for some women: death by freezing, shot by husband, drowned, froze to death, pauper who went 16 days without food and committed suicide, murdered, drowned while in a fit, smallpox, killed by the kick of a horse. I was astounded by the number of Woodbury women who died from scalding, childbirth, and exhaustion. It wasn't specified that any of the women died in childbirth, but there were so many entries like the first one, where the mother died several days after her infant.

The deaths of the children, which by far comprised the majority of the book, were the hardest to read:

October 20, 1711 First-born son of Noah Hinman, 1wk

Dec. 30, 1715 Mary, daughter of Thomas Mallery, after 5 yrs languishing, 9 years

December 11, 1722 John, son of Jeremiah Thomas, killed with a cart

October 16, 1727 John Brownson, died at a dance

July 24, 1747 Sarah, (2nd of that name) dau of John Twiss 1 month

September 24, 1798 Two infant children of Uriel Strong

November 13, 1816 Daughter of Capt. P.F. Peck, drowned age 3

July 26, 1837 Daughter of George Taylor, scalded age 3

February 6, 1844 Colored infant, murdered

Page after page listed *Infant daughter, Infant son, Infant of, Child of, Son of, Daughter of.* The final entry in the book, 219 years later, was just as heartbreaking as the first entry:

December 18, 1897 Earl, son of William Crowell 18 months

And then there were the brief entries, many of the women listed as black, negro, or negress:

1750 Mary, an aged widow

1754 Dorcas, negro servant of Deacon Samuel Minor

1763 Rachael (Ebenezer Talman's negress)

1766 Wife of a Dutchman at the mines

1789 Ginny (negro girl belonging to Roswell Ransom)

I closed my tired eyes, and just as I had done the day before in the town hall, I realized I had time-traveled—not in an Einstein, Stephen Hawking, quantum physics kind of way, but by way of immersion. I found myself so absorbed in what I was uncovering that when I looked up, I blinked my eyes at the overhead fluorescent lights and rows of library computers. I almost resented the fact I had to go home, throw together some sort of dinner, and do lesson plans, because these things were keeping me from my new passion—or, dare I say, *obsession.*

Since the food in the freezer had a diminishing life expectancy, for dinner that night we had a mish-mosh of meats cooked on the grill. We all knew the power outage would have been a lot more unpleasant if it had been February. I shared, "Did you guys know that houses were so cold in colonial days that if a huge fire was built in the fireplace, the sap forced out of the wood by the flames froze into *ice* at the end of the logs?"

Mic, who was crazy about the sultry weather in Puerto Rico, shuddered. I continued, "Basins of water froze if left standing in the bedrooms. Even the urine in the chamber pots froze! And Ehris, you know how we watched *Dr. Zhivago* the other night, and remember the scene when the ink froze in the inkwell? That didn't just happen in Siberia. It happened in New England houses! Kinda puts a blackout in August in perspective, doesn't it?"

"How do you suddenly know all of this stuff?" Mic asked.

"I was reading this old book all day at the library. I'm going back tomorrow to finish it."

"And I bet we're gonna be hearing all about it," Mic predicted.

Pointing to the serving plate on the table, I said, "You know how I just called that a mish-mosh of meat? They ate mostly hotchpots or hashes that were a jumbled-up mix of spoon meat and chopped vegetables. Women cooked things that could basically take care of themselves, because they had so many never-ending chores. Nobody ate roast beef or roasted chicken. And the spoons they ate with—because they didn't use forks—were made of pewter, wood, or horn. Sometimes, they put a huge hotchpot, or a pumpkin stewed whole in its shell and filled with milk, on the table-board, and people ate out of it with long handled spoons or hollow wooden straws."

"Okay," said Mic. "I know it's killing you. What's a table-board?"

"The dinner table was a three-foot wide board that rested on supports, kind of like a saw horse. They called it a table-board, and the thing they covered it with during a meal wasn't a tablecloth, it was a board-cloth. Sometimes they made these tables out of the packing boxes that carried stuff from England to the colonies."

Mic filled his glass with the water Jim had gotten from the firehouse, and I said, "Nobody drank water—they believed water made you sick. They all drank hard cider and ale, even the kids." I picked a pile of notes off the table and said, "I saw this in some other book, and wrote it down. *In 1790, figures showed annual per-capita alcohol consumption for everybody over 15 amounted to 34 gallons of beer and cider, five gallons of distilled spirits, and one gallon of wine.*"

"Yo, I always get mixed up. What's *per capita* mean again?" Mic asked Jim.

"Per person," said Jim. "It means per person."

"Wow, that's a lot a drinkin'," Ehris responded.

"No, it's actually less than a gallon a week per person," Jim calculated. "I bet the average person nowadays drinks half a gallon of soda or something a day, and if they weren't drinking water back then, that's not very much liquid."

"How can you figure that out in your head?" Ehris asked, as she and Mic gave Jim one of their looks. He was always doing these mental statistical calculations.

I shot all three of them a dirty look and said, "Whoa, whoa! You guys rolled your eyes about the frozen sap, the hotch pot, and the noggin. Now you get all excited about...."

"You never said anything about a noggin," Mic interrupted.

"Oh, no, Mic! Now you got her going again," Ehris groaned.

"Well, a noggin was what they drank all the booze out of. It's a small mug or cup. A popular beverage was a quince drink made from hot rum, sugar, and quince preserves. Hey, they also drank out of gourds!" I shouted as my family cleared the table in mock haste and fled the patio.

CHAPTER FIFTY-FOUR

Ehris

My mom and I were watching a Netflix movie a few nights later when I paused it and asked, "So, what special thing do you wanna do for your birthday tomorrow?"

"I was secretly hoping you'd ask me that," she answered.

In a very unsubtle move, she raised her chin and tipped her head at the coffee table where a library paperback entitled *Your Guide to Cemetery Research* was bookmarked with torn pieces of yellow legal paper. It took a few moments before it registered, and then I cried, "Oh, no! You wanna go to the *cemetery*? With *me*?!"

"Well, I was going through more information at the library, and I found out that Solomon and Mary Root are buried in Old North Cemetery. We just have to go in there and find six/D/ten."

"Six/D/ten? What's *that*?"

"I think it's the row and the section. I don't know what the other number means, but like, how hard can it be to find her?"

"Eww. *That's* the special thing you want to do for your birthday?"

"Well, you wanna hear what I'd *really* like to do, but you'll probably think I'm a weirdo?"

"I already think you're a weirdo," I assured her. "So, go ahead."

"Can we get lunch, or something, before we go?"

"And bring it with us? You mean like a *picnic*?! This is like when we were little and you took us to the cemetery with juice boxes and cookies!"

"Oh, that." She waved it away. "I just wanted you guys to try and understand that cemeteries weren't scary places, and that death was just part of life."

"Yeah, but I was like three," I clarified.

"So? You're not three anymore. Can we do it?"

"Okay, I guess...." I said unenthusiastically.

"But you have to act like you're enjoying it when we get there," she insisted.

"Okay, fine. Since it's your birthday, I guess I can't refuse," I agreed.

"Can we do one other thing?"

"What?" I asked suspiciously.

"I think it would be nice if we brought Mary Root a bouquet from some of the flowers we have growing here at the house. Who knows, with some of those old wildflowers, maybe she's the one who transplanted them from the woods and fields."

Six giant oaks stood sentry at Old North Cemetery. With her scribbled notes from *Your Guide to Cemetery Research* and our bag of sandwiches and drinks, my mom was chattering away about how happy she was at the possibility of finding Mary Root's grave, on her birthday, with me. I had picked a bouquet of Queen Anne's lace, daisies, and black-eyed Susans, and tied them with a thin purple ribbon. Its curled ends caught the breeze as I carried the flowers to the cemetery entrance.

My mom merrily informed me that while a fieldstone wall now surrounded the graveyard, "a *living fence* originally encircled the cemetery, and it was made from trees or shrubs, like a hedgerow," she shared. "They planted the bushes six inches apart, and apparently they quickly grew together to keep out predators like wolves. You know that expression of burying someone 'six feet under?' It came about so wild animals couldn't smell a decaying body and dig it up."

"Eww, blech! Wait, I don't get it," I interjected. "Like, what did they do while they were waiting for the shrubs to grow together? It didn't just happen in a few weeks. Like, did they just shrug and say, 'Oh well, in a few years the predators won't be able to get into the cemetery?' But then when the shrubs *did* grow together, couldn't the wolves and stuff just go in the entrance?"

With a reprimanding look, my mom replied, "I'm thinking there was a gate, Ehris. But that's not the point of why we're here."

Huge chunks of white and pink silica topped the massive stone entrance columns. Their simple beauty almost made me forget they were guards at a place of sadness. I realized that before hearses existed, wagons and carriages had entered the cemetery bearing coffins.

About ten steps into Old North Cemetery, we discovered that it wasn't organized by sections or rows. Actually, it didn't seem organized at all. The names on many of the weather-worn headstones were impossible to read from the ravages of time. Most of the markers were scabbed with fungus and lichen. The cemetery wasn't neglected, but we had entered at a point where there were many crumbled and illegible tombstones. Exposed mountain laurel roots strangled some of the broken chunks, like the tightly wrapped coils of a boa constrictor squeezing the life out of its prey.

My mom said, "You can't believe all the stuff I found online about easier ways to read the gravestones. It's very controversial, but now I get it."

"How would reading a gravestone be *controversial?*" I asked.

"There was actually an entire website about headstone engravings. I guess there are lots of people who hang out in cemeteries and try to read the inscriptions on the oldest stones," she explained.

"You should have gotten one of them to come here with you. I'm sure they would have enjoyed your birthday picnic plan," I quipped.

"The website said the best way to read them is to wet the stone, then cover part of it with shaving cream, and then scrape off the excess with a piece of Styrofoam. The shaving cream fills in the depressions, and then the white letters appear in contrast on the stone."

I asked sarcastically, "Who would have a chunk of Styrofoam just hanging around for the one day they go to the cemetery?"

"Okay, it gets better, because you're supposed to take along a big jug of water to wash off the shaving cream."

"Sandwiches, drinks, Styrofoam, shaving cream, water jugs—the perfect picnic!"

"So that's where the big controversy is," my mom jabbered. "A lot of people say it's not a good idea to use shaving cream on gravestones, because they're porous and there's chemicals and greasy stuff in the shaving cream that get stuck in all the grooves and damages the stone."

"Well, then every headstone in here must have been shaving creamed, because they all look pretty messed up," I noted.

"The website actually had this whole analysis of shaving cream today and shaving cream from forty years ago. It said old shaving cream contained chemicals, which was bad for the stones, and modern-day shaving cream contains skin softening stuff that appeals to bacteria, fungus, and mold, which also messes up the stones."

"Maybe you should just tell Daddy all this the next time he's shaving. I can't believe we're in a cemetery on your birthday talking about shaving cream!" I exclaimed.

"One person on the website said she uses Cool Whip instead of shaving cream."

"Great, more stuff for your picnic."

"Another guy said just getting the stone wet can make the carvings stand out and he said you should bring along several gallons of water. And another guy said you just need those foil car sun shades to use like a reflector to bounce light on the stone from just the right angle."

"You'd need a cart to carry all that stuff around the cemetery," I sighed as we wandered around, trying to make out the inscriptions on the headstones.

Velya

Spending time in a graveyard can teach you a lot about living. As I stopped at each grave, I swear I could almost hear the silent stories of perfect strangers. In a way, though, they didn't feel like perfect strangers, since I had met many of these people in the little *Barnes' Mortality* book at the library. Many of the headstones were grouped together closely and haphazardly, like a family, with the taller stones for the adults. It was the tiniest stones of the babies, many of them tilted, sunken, or broken, that were the saddest to read. Husbands and wives had certain positioning in the grave. Today, we stack coffins on top of each other, but back then, a wife was placed to her husband's left in the grave. A bride stands to the groom's left for the same reason. It all came from the belief that woman was created from the left side, the rib of Adam.

"That's the Galpins' baby," I said to Ehris, pointing to a small flat stone marked 1678 with the name Esther. "Her mother died eight days later—see, she's right there. Her name was Esther, too. I remember sitting in the library and thinking about the poor husband. And there's Submit Cooper. I remember her, too," I said as we passed a stone that was relatively easy to read. "All of her kids died in the smallpox epidemic of 1770. I read about smallpox after I saw so many people here had died from it. Did you know that in like 1050 A.D., there was a Buddhist nun who ground up scabs taken from people infected with smallpox into a powder, and then blew it into the nostrils of healthy people?"

"Eww, that's really gross! How many scabs do you need to be able to grind them up into a powder? But it's pretty cool if it worked, like the first smallpox vaccine."

"Yeah, exactly. I think the actual smallpox vaccine wasn't invented until almost 1800. So just think—Submit's kids only missed it by 30 years."

We had barely covered a quarter of the cemetery. It was very slow going, and several times, we thought we spotted Mary Root's name; but they were all false alarms. Ehris and I decided to split up so we could cover more ground. As much as Ehris had grumbled about being here, I noticed she carefully bent to read each headstone, sometimes pausing before she moved to the next one.

Back and forth Ehris and I wandered, making sure to check every single grave. Usually, the woman's headstone was smaller than her husband's, and many of the first names conveyed the submissive roles they played: Comfort, Thankful, Mercy, Temperance, Charity.

"I don't understand some of this," Ehris called. "Some of these phrases are so weird."

"Like what?" I asked.

"Like this one. I think it says he was *casually killed by the fall of an oak*. What's so casual about a tree falling on you?"

"I think *casually* back then meant accidentally. I just saw one back there that said a guy was *casually shot*. You know how some insurance companies are still called fire and casualty? It's just an example of how language changes. There was a woman over in that section who was called a *relict*, and I'm pretty sure that means she was a widow."

"The really old ones are pretty creepy with the skulls, and bones, and skeletons carved at the top."

"All the ones I saw like that were the slate stones." I said. "Those, and the fieldstone ones, are the oldest. Well, actually, that's not true. The earliest markers were made of wood, but those rotted away, obviously. I think the skeletons were a symbol of mortality. If you see any with a severed branch or a candle flame, it's supposed to mean the person's life was cut short or it was snuffed out."

"I saw a few that had faces with wings. I guess that's supposed to be about their soul flying away," Ehris said.

We only had a small section left to explore, and I was starting to get discouraged. "I'm getting worried, Ehris. What if Mary Root has one of those headstones that are just impossible to read? We may have passed right over her."

"Don't worry. If she's in here, we'll find her. No picnic until we do," she teased.

Ehris and I met up at the far end of the cemetery. Neither of us had found Mary Root, or any member of the Minor family. Disappointed, I sighed. "Well, I guess the only thing I can do is go back to the library and see if I can find the names of some of the other people buried near six/D/ten. Then maybe we'll see a name we recognize from today, and we can try and figure out how this row-and-section system works, if there even *is* a system. This really sucks, though. It would have been the best birthday present if we had found her."

"We can go over to the library now, if you want," Ehris offered.

Pointing to a granite headstone, I said, "Look at that one over there, Ehris. It's backwards. The writing on all the other ones in that section faces Main Street. This one looks down the hill. Did you read that one? I totally missed it."

The headstone was, indeed, facing in a different direction than all the others around it. I was hoping against hope as I hurried over to it. A scraggly sumac tree grew to one side of the erect headstone, which stood all by itself. I knew I'd found her.

"Ehris!" I shouted. "This is her! I know it." Approaching the stone from the rear, I circled around to the front. With my left hand resting on top of the gray stone, I dared to look at the inscription. There were no mortality symbols cut into the round-shouldered stone, just the basic facts: name, death date, and age—the CliffsNotes version of a life.

Here Lyes Interred

Mary Root Minor wife of Solomon who dyed July 28,

1791 In her 38th Year entered into rest

"We did it! We did it!" I cried, grabbing Ehris in a hug. "We found her!"

"*You* found her," she corrected. "It's pretty weird we were just about to give up."

"This is going to sound totally fake, but it's like something was telling me to look over at this stone. We searched right here. How'd we miss it the first time?"

"Why is this the only one that faces down the hill? And the engraving is so clear, it looks perfect," Ehris observed.

"I was getting so freaked out when we saw all those ruined ones!"

"Oh, no," Ehris said, looking me in the eyes. "Are you going to cry?"

"Not yet, we have to take a picture first."

"A *picture*? You brought your *camera* to the cemetery?"

"Well, yeah, of course I did," I answered, opening the lunch bag and pulling out my small black camera case. "You think it's okay if I touch the headstone while you take the photo? I mean like that's not disrespectful, right?"

"I'm sure it's fine," Ehris said, and snapped some photos.

"I am *so* happy! This is like the best birthday present I've ever gotten! Can you believe we found her? Wait until we bring Daddy and Mic here. Oh, man, Ehris, thank you so, so much for coming here with me. That's the icing on the cake—we found her together!"

Ehris placed the bouquet she had gathered at the base of Mary Root's headstone, and we both stood quietly for a few moments. We had driven the road her grave overlooked countless times, yet never suspected she had been laid to rest at the top of the hill.

"It's not very level here for us to sit and eat," I said. "Should we go over there by the woods where it's flat to have our lunch?"

"You would have eaten on top of her grave if it *was* level?"

"Uhh…yeah…probably. Why? Is that weird? But that's okay, we don't have to," I reassured Ehris as we walked over to a grassy patch of lawn and sat down. "You know, sometimes things seem perfectly normal to me, like eating over there with Mary Root. But judging by your reaction, I guess it's not…."

After she handed me my chicken salad sandwich and unwrapped her veggie burger, Ehris said, "I just think it's creepy. I don't think it's a bad thing."

The graves in this cemetery were so old, it must have been at least 100 years since a funeral had taken place here. The rituals involved with burying the dead had changed. In the past, it had been family and friends who performed the activities associated with death. From building the coffin, to washing and dressing the deceased person, to digging the grave, death was dealt with on a more personal basis. Today, we pay other people to do these tasks.

I said, "You know I'm going to tell you the interesting stuff about death and dying that was in the book on the coffee table, right? I waited until you were finished eating—give me credit for that, at least."

"I knew that was coming. Okay, I guess I'm ready," Ehris said, screwing the cap back on her stainless steel water bottle.

Without even asking, she handed me my yellow legal pad full of scribbly notes. I took a considerable amount of teasing from my family about my unbridled enthusiasm and kookiness, but despite their protests, I noticed they all stuck around. My theory was, as long as *you* know you're nutty, you're probably okay.

"When a person was close to death, family and friends would gather for the death watch. They usually announced the death by bell-ringing to frighten away evil spirits, and also to spread the word. I saw one little mention somewhere about some kind of cookies called 'death cakes' that were handed out to let people know someone had died."

"Wait, so what did it say on the cookies? If they were just blank, it would be like, 'Okay, someone died, but we don't know who it was.' Like, did they write 'Marge died' or 'R.I.P. Arthur' on every cookie?"

"I have no idea what they put on the cookies, Ehris!"

Ehris continued, "Remember, in Brazil, how the car with the loudspeaker would drive around the streets and announce when someone had died?"

"I forgot all about that. I do remember Isabela being shocked when I told her that people who die in Connecticut in the middle of the winter usually aren't buried until spring, and they store the body somewhere. In colonial days, when the winters were really bad, they sometimes had to wait until the spring thaw to dig the grave, and they stored the body in the barn or somewhere."

"*Blechhh!* Imagine Aunt Abigail being stored in your toolshed all winter?"

I explained, "Undertakers weren't used until about 1850, and before that, it was family members and neighbors who prepared the body for burial. If a woman died in childbirth, the midwife was one of the people who helped. It was always women in early America who handled everything involving a burial, just like it was women who delivered all the babies. But when male undertakers and obstetricians got into the act, the women were forced out," I said with disgust.

Ehris huffed, "How come some men think they can do things better than women? It's so annoying!"

"They had to work pretty quickly before *rigor mortis* set in. They wanted to give the dead person the appearance of sleeping, so their arms were folded across the chest, their feet were tied together, and they placed coins on the eyelids to keep them shut."

"They tied their feet together? Did they think they were going to move?" Ehris joked.

Ignoring her, I continued, "Then they tied a cord or kerchief under the chin and over the head to keep the mouth from dropping open."

"Did they have open coffins? Because the cord under their chin and coins on their eyelids would kind of ruin the look of the person sleeping," Ehris said sarcastically.

"They buried them in their best clothes or a shroud," I said.

"Okay, cool," Ehris said, trying to cut me off. "Can we take a break for cupcakes?"

"Ehris, you crack me up! You act like I'm an annoying weirdo!"

"But you are!"

I studied Ehris as she nibbled her cupcake. Her ballerina

collarbones and the magic of her Gibson girl hair, which was piled atop her head in a soft bouffant style, exuded effortlessness and made me wonder, yet again, *how in the world did I create half of this*? I thought about how lucky I was to have her. For a time, she and I had shared the same body. Love was too weak a word for what I felt for her.

"All this cemetery stuff makes me think even more about what jerks Jose and Grandpa are, and it gets me *so* mad," Ehris revealed. "People back then actually had something to complain about, but today, they don't; they're just evil. When I see people out with their grandparents, it makes me sad, like I could be bringing Nazey to the movies or just hanging out with her. And then I think about how nice Guilherme and Zoe were to us in Brazil, and how I just want to see them again."

I nodded. Nodded and cradled my amazing child, who had gone through so much. Trying to get her to laugh, I said, "Did you know, it took six bushels of ashes and twenty-four pounds of grease to make a barrel of soap?"

We were both a blubbering mess, and as we held each other, I asked, "Do you think we're healing?"

"I think we're starting to," Ehris said as I brushed her hair away from her face.

"This is the last thing I want to tell you, and then we can go home," I said to Ehris. "The colonists had lots of superstitions. They stopped the clocks at the time of death so everyone knew what time the person had died, and then they started the clocks again after the burial to symbolize the family starting a new period in their life."

I slipped my notes back into our lunch bag and put my hand out to Ehris. She helped me up from the spot beneath the sumac tree. At the exact same time, we each placed a hand on Mary Root's headstone, as if in farewell.

"That one about the clocks is kind of nice, the symbolism and all that," Ehris said, nodding approvingly.

"Okay, you're going to think I'm getting all schmaltzy, but maybe the 'starting the clocks again' idea is sort of the same for us. We're a family starting a new period in our lives, too."

"I *do* think you're schmaltzy, but I guess you're allowed to be on your birthday," conceded Ehris as we held hands and walked to the car.

CHAPTER FIFTY-FIVE

Ehris

Our Bridgewater house had had so much shade, we'd never been able to have a garden. At our new house, I was finally able to have the vegetable garden I'd always wanted. With only organic and heirloom seeds, I grew cherry tomatoes, kale, cucumbers, radishes, leeks, lettuce, squash, and sunflowers. My dad built me raised wooden planting beds, which we filled with four truckloads of horse manure shoveled from our neighbor's farm. In the Vitamix blender, I concocted homemade insect repellents from garlic, chili powder, and dish soap. The garden was my therapy, and I spent many peaceful hours building twig arbors and harvesting the bounty.

One afternoon in early fall, I was picking lipstick-red cherry tomatoes. There were hundreds of them, and I wanted to get them all picked before the first frost. The monotonous movements gave me time to think about healing. My dad wasn't opening his heart, so he wasn't healing. My mom's research about colonial women was bringing her back to life. I realized that there were two ways I could respond to my heartbreak—either react with bitterness like my dad, or start to transform my suffering into a creative force, like my mom.

I was raised in a family passionate about holistic medicine. For all of my growing-up years, I remember my mom giving me arnica pellets whenever I fell down. Kids thought I was a weirdo when I ate my Ezekiel bread sandwiches in the cafeteria. We had all been following the Blood Type Diet since I was nine years old, and none of us consumed corn syrup, wheat, or pasteurized milk. We didn't use a microwave or drink out of plastic water bottles. When people came over and saw my kombucha, kimchi, and kefir fermenting on the counter, they said things like "Yuck! Gross! That looks like a science fair project gone wrong!"

At age 16, I asked for (and received) a dehydrator and a Vitamix for my birthday. When my parents and I declined my Gardasil vaccine, my health teacher proclaimed, "Your mom is being very irresponsible." I became interested in Reiki in middle school, and attained Reiki Master certification at age 17.

After freshman year, when I left Shepaug Valley High School to finish school online, my parents were told that I would become a "social outcast" and "never get into college" (I actually graduated college a semester early). After I was diagnosed with West Nile virus as a teenager, an infectious disease specialist nonchalantly stated, "You'll never get the virus out of your system." Six months later, blood tests revealed that castor oil packs had drawn it out of my liver and body, and I was virus-free.

People critically judge the natural world. Drinking raw milk or refusing a flu shot is considered radical, but popping antidepressants with side effects like suicidal thoughts isn't questioned. Using a menstrual cup, taking fermented cod liver oil, and smudging are seen as strange. Most people believe that healing cancer without chemotherapy and radiation is impossible. But allowing someone to slice open your chest and graft your leg veins into your heart is considered normal and conservative.

I delved deeper into my herb garden, and the perfumed walk became a mystical part of my world. Even the coldest winter eventually transforms into a field of green, flowers, and new life. The wise words in old herbal remedy books written by my healer foremothers brought me comfort. I felt empowered to stop being a broken heart.

Our naturopath, Liz Herman, suggested to my mom and me that with all the emotional junk we were going through, we should try flower essences. We had never heard of them, but as we sat on the floor of the health food store that afternoon digging through the *Flower Essence Repertory,* I felt the new way of healing pollinate my mind.

Flower essences, which are *not* essential oils, are made from the flowering parts of plants. Taken internally, they uniquely address the emotional and mental aspects of wellness without side effects. There are hundreds of flower essences for issues like stress, grief, shock, indecision, anger, and body image. After reading about patterns of imbalance and the positive qualities of various essences, we chose Agrimony and White Chestnut for my mom, and Star of Bethlehem and Rock Water for me. Agrimony helps people who hide their pain behind a cheerful face, and White Chestnut is for those who can't prevent unwanted thoughts from entering their minds. Star of Bethlehem softens shock and trauma, and Rock Water is for self-denial and rigidity.

Almost immediately, my mom began sleeping more soundly. Before White Chestnut, her thoughts, especially at bedtime, would circle round and round in her head like a looped recording. I noticed that the heartbreak in her eyes seemed lessened. Star of Bethlehem eased my emotional whiplash, while Rock Water permitted me to let loose and have fun. When I relented and finally let my mom buy me a pair of high-heeled gray above-the-knee suede boots, I knew I had stopped punishing myself for something that had been out of my control and wasn't even my fault.

CHAPTER FIFTY-SIX

Velya

On the first chilly night of the year, we lit the woodstove, and Ehris brewed a pot of tea from the lemon balm in her garden. Over dinner, I went back to my history lessons, telling everyone that the coffee in colonial times was often made from parched rye and chestnuts.

"After the Boston Tea Party, they came up with their own homegrown tea substitutes made out of goldenrod, raspberry leaves, and ribwort—whatever that is. They made *liberty tea* out of four-leaved loosestrife, and I read about one little girl who was served tea—real tea—at someone's house, and she threw her teacup out the window and said she only drank liberty tea," I laughed.

"Well, I wouldn't have minded drinking *this* tea," Jim said, raising his cup to Ehris.

"I've been waiting to tell you guys this other stuff, because I guarantee you're going to make fun of me and I'm not going to hear the end of it."

"Like what?" Ehris asked.

"Okay, well, remember this is all according to that book. It said the seas, rivers, and lakes teemed with fish, and in New York Bay, up until the 1800s, there were five- and six-foot lobsters."

"That would be like Daddy walking around with lobster claws!" exclaimed Mic as he made lobster claw motions with his hands.

This joke was aimed directly at me. Whenever I tried to picture measurements in my head, I always used Jim's height as a point of reference. Mic and Ehris had grown up hearing me say, "That couch would be equal to one and a half Daddys," or "Picture Daddy standing on top of Daddy, and that would be twelve feet."

"The book said the foot-long ones 'were better for the table,'" I said.

"What's that mean?" Ehris asked. "Were they better *tasting*, or did they just *fit* on the table better? Oh, sorry, I mean the table-board."

"How come every time we have a dinner table conversation, it goes off in five million directions, and I am the butt of all the jokes?" I asked.

As usual, no one answered.

"In Brooklyn, it was common to catch foot-long oysters," I continued.

"How hard was it to catch a foot-long oyster? Like, really, how fast can a foot-long oyster even move? They couldn't just dart away!" Ehris retorted.

"I saw a show about oysters on National Geographic," Jim said. "They have clear blood."

"Oh, my god, can we get back to the colonists?" I begged. "Here's the one where you're all gonna be rolling on the floor. Did you know that in Virginia, rivers were so full of fish that horses crossing the river stepped on them and killed them?"

They all just looked at me. Then Mic stood up, imitated a horse crossing a river, and said, "Can't you just picture the horses picking up their hooves and saying, 'Oops, there's another one! Oops, there's *another* one!'"

Learning all this colonial stuff was the springboard behind my next preoccupation. In our kitchen, there was a black woodstove we had never used. The woodstove sat on the wide-board floor, and behind it was a brick wall and wooden mantle where I displayed two antique spice cabinets we had lugged home from Slovakia. As a history nut and antique lover, I just *knew* that behind all that brick was some sort of really old fireplace, and the thought gnawed away at me.

I sensed that an activity could be therapeutic for Jim, who thrived when engaged in unusual projects. That night at dinner, after discussing the foot-long oysters and the Jim-sized lobsters, I purposefully said, "In the whole eight months we've lived here, I've always had a feeling there's something cool behind that woodstove in the kitchen."

That was all it took. Within minutes, we had left the dinner table, and Jim started some exploratory investigating. He pulled off the stove's vent pipe, then grabbed a flashlight and hurried to the basement. Within ten minutes, he had brought up an assortment of sledgehammers, pry bars, and crowbars, and the demolition began. We were so psyched to begin that we didn't even take the time to hang drop cloths. It didn't take too long to crash through the bricks—though I was working the camera, not the hammers—and once the dust settled (all over the kitchen!), we discovered a solid fieldstone and cement wall.

Jim, the construction expert, said, "This isn't original to the house. It looks like it's from the 1950s."

"Oh man, that's so cool!" I cried enthusiastically. "That means there's gotta be something behind that wall!"

The demolition continued.

CHAPTER FIFTY-SEVEN

Velya

Jim came home the next morning with a rented jackhammer. There probably aren't too many women who have had weekend jackhammer work done in their kitchen, but I took it in stride since, after all, it *had* been my bright idea. For some reason, we still hadn't hung any drop cloths. To add to the craziness, in a week, we were hosting a huge party to thank all the people who had helped us since we had returned from Brazil.

The thing that motivated us and compensated for the sheer filth of this job was the fact that we knew something really incredible was behind the stone wall. Every time we dislodged a good-sized rock, we'd shine a flashlight around.

"Look!" Mic screamed. "There's a huge fireplace back there! The kind you can stand up in!"

Lying on his back and shining the flashlight through a hole in the cement, grimy Jim announced, "I think there's a beehive oven, too!"

We all took turns with the sledgehammers. Dripping sweat left tracks in the colonial soot that covered our faces. When we took a lunch break, I pulled little pieces of cement and stone from my cleavage. I took a look at Jim and snorted,

"Oh, man, you look just like Mary Poppins' boyfriend—the chimney sweep guy. What was his name again?"

"I have *no* idea what you're talking about," he said through gritty gritted teeth. "You're so funny, Wifely."

"Jim, you're not fooling me. You're more excited than anyone about this. Ehris, come on! What was the boyfriend's name?" I prodded. "This is going to drive me nuts if I don't remember."

"I don't know. I don't think I ever actually saw the movie." Ehris shrugged.

"I hate when this happens! Now this is gonna be stuck in my head until I remember it!" I grumbled. Two hours later, swinging the sledgehammer, I cried, "Bert! Bert! His name was Bert!"

It took two entire days. Jim estimated that we had removed 3,000 pounds of brick, rock, cement, and paneling. By the time we finished, we had exposed an eight-foot-wide, three-foot-deep, five-foot-high fireplace with baking oven. We found a petrified colonial rat skeleton (it sounded more thrilling when we said it was a colonial rat), antique square-cut nails, and a large iron swinging crane for hanging kettles and pots. In amazement, we constantly asked each other, "Why in the world would someone have covered this up?"

All four of us could fit inside the fireplace and look up the massive sooty chimney at blue sky, and later, the stars. As I gazed at those stars hundreds and thousands of light years away, I realized I was also looking far back into time.

Once all the rubble had been lugged outside and we had vacuumed up some of the mess with a Shop-Vac, Jim started prying off the last of the wood paneling and announced, "We have king's wood under here!" Sure enough, above the fireplace were very old wooden boards, and several of them were over 24 inches wide. Jim had worked on other old houses, so we had all heard about king's wood and were familiar with its history.

By the 17th century, England had depleted its forests and was in need of tall, straight timber for its wooden ships, especially the masts. Since all of New England was Crown land, the king took control of the tallest and greatest of these trees, most of them eastern white pine. Each year, usually in the winter, representatives of the king would mark these trees with hatchet marks, and it was illegal for them to be cut and used by anyone but the Royal British Navy.

The colonists were understandably upset, and many rebelled. Of course, the Revolutionary War wasn't fought over just one issue, but some colonists felt that being denied the use of the trees was as unjust as the tea and stamp tax. The pine-tree flag was one of the flags used during the American Revolution. It featured a pine tree with the motto "An Appeal to Heaven."

"Holy smoke!" I cheered. "This just keeps getting better and better!"

Mic said, "So it looks like whoever built this house was a little rebellious!"

"Up until the Revolution, it was definitely illegal to have this wood," Jim agreed, running his hand over the boards. "I don't know about you guys, but I've had it for tonight. I cannot move one more rock."

"I feel like my arms are going to fall off," Ehris agreed.

"Well, let's leave everything just like it is," I said. "My legs are so tired I don't know if I'm walking on my feet or my ankles. We'll finish up all the cleaning in the morning."

Even with my short, choppy hair, it took three rounds of shampoo to get all the crud out of my scalp. As Jim snored away, I noticed with interest that the lines in his forehead looked less like a freshly furrowed field.

CHAPTER FIFTY-EIGHT

Velya

Jordan suggested I push myself in my writing and memories, and go even deeper outside of my comfort zone. And so, like Karen Blixen, Meryl Streep's character in the 1985 film *Out of Africa*, I did just that.

In 1913, Karen Blixen entered a marriage of convenience and moved to Africa. Her husband turned out to be a womanizer and she contracted syphilis from him, leaving her unable to have children. She went home to Denmark for treatment, and when she returned to Africa, she fell madly in love with Denys Finch Hatton (Robert Redford's character); who, she eventually learned, she could not own or tame, just as she could not tame Africa. After years of hard work, her coffee plantation finally yielded a bountiful harvest, only to be destroyed by fire. Out of money, her love affair with Denys over, she arranged to sell everything she owned and leave Africa. The last time she saw Denys, she was alone in her empty house and said to him, "I've got this little thing that I've learned to do lately. When it gets so bad...and I think I can't go on...I try to make it worse. I make myself think about our camp on the river...and the first time you took me flying. How good it all was. And when I'm certain that I can't stand it…I go one moment more. And then I know I can bear anything. Would you like to help me?"

"Yes," he responded.

"Come dance with me then."

Like Karen Blixen, there was one memory so painful that it actually made my heart hurt when I forced myself to replay it.

Growing up, Jordan and I, and the kids down the road, all walked the half mile to our bus stop and back home again in the afternoon. We never thought much of it—actually, it was a fun time to fool around. On rainy days, our mother usually piled all of us into the station wagon and drove to the bus stop, and was there waiting in the afternoon. Once in a while, a neighbor named Mrs. Gray picked us up, but invariably complained that we slammed her car door too hard and predicted we would eventually knock the door off its hinges. Even in elementary school, we realized this was baloney, and imitated her as soon as we hopped out of the car. Sometimes, in rainy weather, our mother couldn't drive us, and sent us off with embarrassing umbrellas. Actually, they were just normal black umbrellas, but carrying one compromised the tomboy image I had fought so hard to achieve. As soon as we reached the bus stop, I always stashed mine behind a huge limestone boulder, planning to retrieve it when we walked home. I always forgot it, probably on purpose, but my mother seemed to have a never-ending umbrella supply.

Finally, one day when I was about ten, my mother went a little crazy and warned me she had had it with me losing umbrellas. Actually, she gave her infamous "had it up to here" speech in which she made a karate-chop motion at her throat while simultaneously shouting, "I've had it up to here with you leaving umbrellas at the bus stop!" Early on, I had astutely noticed that during these monologues when she'd "had it up to here," her hand never went higher than her throat. This time, though, she seemed pretty serious.

We grew up in a waterfront house on Rainbow Lake. Life was dictated by the seasons, and winter was an amazing time. There were years the lake stayed frozen all winter, and we were able to walk home from the bus stop on the ice. Instead of reenacting scenes from *The Wizard of Oz*, as we did when we walked home on the road, we pretended to be ice-skating characters from *Hans Brinker*. There was an occasional year when it would get very cold for an extended period without a lot of wind or snow, and we could skate all the way across the smooth, frozen lake. Sometimes, the ice was so clear we could see fish swimming below. As the temperature fluctuated in the morning or evening, the ice expanded or contracted, resulting in a frozen lake chant from deep below. We grew up listening to the voice of the ice.

While my best friend, Lizzie, and I prepared for the Olympics in white figure skates sporting little jingle bells and homemade yarn pom-poms, Jordan and the other boys played ice hockey at every opportunity. This was ice hockey without helmets, pads, or parental supervision, but boys of all ages were included. More hours were probably spent shoveling the "rink" than actually playing. All of the hockey sticks were bandaged with layers of black electrician's tape snatched from garage workshops or dusty basement shelves. But that didn't muffle the *smack* as puck met stick and the crack-slap ricocheted off Pine Mountain and across Rainbow Lake. It was an evocative noise, as was the cutting, scraping, ringing sound of the hockey skates—a crisp, clean sound as the steel edges of the skates dug into the ice. There could be 20 kids out on the ice—but somehow, it was an *alone* sound, not a *lonely* sound. It had something to do with the oddly omnipotent feeling of gliding over places where I had swum just months before, yet always, there was the lurking danger of skating on thin ice.

One Saturday in the year of the umbrella admonition, we experienced one of those glorious ice-like-glass periods. My mother brought a blanket down from the house. Jordan, my father, my mother, and I each held a corner as we skated onto the ice. The wind quickly caught the blanket and we flew effortlessly across the ice, the rush of wind in our faces.

The blanket idea was such a brilliant one that someone in the family got the idea to try it with umbrellas. With the blanket as a sail, we zipped across the ice, and merely had to drop the corners in order to stop. However, it was impossible to close the wind-filled umbrellas as we flew, unable to steer. The rest of my family let go of their umbrellas. Suddenly, I found myself alone on the ice with the black umbrella dragging me down the center of the lake, heading towards the dam. My parents and Jordan were shouting at me from shore and making frantic flailing arm gestures. I knew if I let go of the umbrella it would be lost, and I'd be in big trouble. Little did I know they were screaming for me to "Drop the umbrella!"

The dam was a place we always knew to avoid when row-boating, turtle hunting, or skating. It held a scary fascination, as we knew danger existed not only in going over the dam, but also in being caught in the backwash below the dam. Everything seemed to be in slow motion as I actually pictured myself, black umbrella in hand, going over the dam, kind of like a crashing Mary Poppins. I glanced to my left, and running parallel to me on the shore was my father in heavy black boots. I had probably traveled a quarter of a mile by then, and he was racing through the woods and yelling something. Finally, I heard him holler through cupped hands, "Honey, drop the umbrella!"

He must have been exhausted, but he carried me all the way home. The feeling of being rescued by my father was indescribable. I still remember the way his scratchy jacket smelled. How his boots scuffed along the ice, and how the sound changed when he reached the woods. The way I kind of bobbed up and down as he walked. Though I was probably ten years old, I remembered feeling the way I used to when I was little and sat on his lap to watch *Johnny Yuma* and *Ben Casey*. It always felt as if it were very, very late at night, and I was participating in something grown-up and special.

Like Karen Blixen, I pushed myself one memory further, and then I knew I could bear anything. I remembered how protected I had felt as we watched TV together—the way his hand, resting on my shoulder, made a warm spot that suddenly turned cold, as if something were missing, when he removed it to eat a Cheese Nip from the wooden snack bowl or take a drink of soda.

My father had made a choice he would be forced to live with. He had alienated me in the process, but not seeing him wasn't the same as forgetting him. It didn't mean my memory banks had been erased, like those of an obsolete robot.

How good I thought it all was. But as Jordan once told me, "Maybe you never really knew them, and they just existed for you as hope of what they could be, or what you wanted them to be." Like the crashing Mary Poppins, it's water over the dam. Yet as long as there's someone around to remember it, a memory still exists. Under the pseudonym of Isak Dinesen, Karen Blixen became an author and storyteller. She wrote about her experiences in Africa, yet never returned there. A broken heart does that to you. It hurts too much to go back.

CHAPTER FIFTY-NINE

Velya

❋

The good thing about being messed up for a while is that you can come out of it seeing very clearly. I used to live life anticipating calamities and thinking of worst-case scenarios. I kept all of our income tax returns dating back to the Reagan administration in fear of being audited, and took great pride in the fact that I could find the manuals for all of our appliances in the event of the hot-water heater conking out and flooding the basement. I saved all of my notebooks from graduate school so I could analyze a Shakespearean sonnet at a moment's notice. I rationed my beloved Chanel No. 5 in case something terrible happened and I couldn't afford to buy more. I had certain dish towels earmarked as the "good" dish towels—and never used them. *Good* dish towels?

All the planning, organizing, and worrying didn't prevent disaster from striking, however. When my life was swept away by a tsunami of crap and I had no real control over things, I let go. I allowed myself to be tossed around by the waves until all the debris washed ashore and the water became less murky. You can spend your days creeping around trying to hide from disaster, but then you just end up with a pile of pristine dish towels and a life you missed out on. Disaster—the sort of disaster that leaves you numb on a park bench in Brazil or aching for your husband to come back to you—can be a freaky thing of beauty. Tsunamis reshape the Earth, and our tsunami reshaped me. It may have briefly swallowed me up, but I refused to drown.

It was our vet who made me realize that Ehris and I had healed each other.

Harry, our poor cat Harry, traveled with us to Brazil, and became a little psycho after encountering the stealthy six-foot long dark green lizards that flicked their forked tongues and sunned themselves in the tall grass behind our stucco house. Back in Connecticut after his South American adventure, Harry continued his tomcat ways. The tips of his battle-scarred ears looked like the lacey paper doilies under bake-sale brownies. Despite the fact that he was neutered, his testosterone level still must have been high, because it wasn't unusual for him to roam around for a few days, then come home with scratches and minor injuries.

One day, Harry came home with a patch of skin ripped from his front shoulder. By the time I figured out what was wrong, it had abscessed. The night before our trip to the vet, it opened up. Copious amounts of rust-colored blood and foul-smelling pus, the color and viscosity of chicken gravy, flowed out like a river.

Dr. Elwell shaved Harry and clipped the torn skin away, leaving a dime-sized hole where you could look in and see muscles and connective tissue. When the procedure was finished, I popped Harry back into the cardboard cat carrier and did that clever folding flap trick to keep the box securely closed. Within seconds, his head poked through the center of the folded box top, and like a flower emerging in one of those time-lapse nature videos. The four petals of the box bloomed, and Harry popped out. As I put unhappy Harry back into the box a second time, Dr. Elwell instructed, "Cats heal from the inside out, so don't cover the wound in any way. You'll have to hold him down and press on the abscess to make the pus come out. We don't want the skin healing over the wound too quickly. If it closes prematurely, the risk of recurrence increases. When you clean the wound, gently massage the skin surrounding it with a warm washcloth to open it up and promote drainage."

On the drive home, all 11 of Harry's paws poked through the nickel-sized air holes as he yowled and cried indignantly. That night, I got a warm washcloth ready and cornered Harry in the kitchen. He was surprisingly agreeable as I pressed on his abscess, and pink-tinted pus oozed out. That's when I got my *aha!* moment. Harry's abscess and Jim's refusal to talk about Brazil and his feelings were one and the same. Jim's anger at Jose, and himself, was festering like a sore, juicy pimple.

It's just a matter of time before a throbbing zit explodes with a force that blasts pus onto the bathroom mirror like a tiny Jackson Pollock painting and makes you wonder, *where did all that gunk come from? How long has it been lurking in there, just below the surface?* The experience is undeniably satisfying. That's when you know the worst is over, and the healing process can begin.

Commiserating and resurrecting with Ehris had lanced my purulent abscess and allowed it to drain. Unlike Jim, I hadn't let a scab form too quickly. I didn't just slap a Band-Aid on the issues' infected tissues and pretend they weren't there. I couldn't heal Jim. I knew that when he was ready, and only when he was ready, would he find the strength to open his wound, stick his hand inside like an oncologist performing surgery, pull out the cancerous memories holding him in the past, and make peace with them. But it had to come from within. I couldn't do this for him. All I could do was wait for him. You can only remake your own future, not someone else's.

I was able to look at the entire Jose situation differently than Jim. To Jim, a man's strength was measured by the care he took of those under his protection: his wife, his children. Jim lived by a code of honor.

I blamed Jose.

Jim blamed himself.

Betrayal involves broken trust, and I have no doubt the thought of murdering Jose crossed his mind many times. It's only natural to want to avoid painful memories and feelings, but the more Jim tried to numb himself and push memories away, the worse he seemed to get. As Ehris and I slowly got better, Jim pulled away to the point where it got in the way of our family life. It took a heavy toll. It was hard to understand why Jim wouldn't open up to us—why he was so closed off. He didn't seem angry. The best way to describe it was an emotional numbness. I knew it was important to be patient and understanding. Deep down, I knew it didn't have anything to do with me or our relationship, but frankly, there were days when I just wanted to punch him in the head and say, "Get over it! *We're* not the ones who swindled you. We're trying, and you're not!"

The best parts of Jim had died—or, if they hadn't died, the best parts of him weren't exactly alive anymore. One night, he whimpered in his sleep. *Jim* and *whimper* never would have appeared in the same sentence before Jose's betrayal. I nudged him and said, "Jim, wake up, you're having a nightmare."

"I know," he monotoned. "I dreamed I was trying to kill a guy. I met him on the street. He stole our money."

The reason Jim and I had to heal differently was because the emotion that broke our hearts differed. I think sadness broke my heart—sadness that our family's dream had been shattered. For Jim, it was more about trust and the expectation that Jose would never hurt or betray us. Because Jim was an honorable man who always kept his word, he had trusted Jose to do the same. Back in the 1990s, just like everyone else, I had read the bestselling book about the fundamental psychological differences between the genders, *Men Are from Mars, Women are from Venus*. I understood that the needs of men and women are different, and we also have different ways of dealing with stress or asking for what we need.

Men expect women to think and behave like men, and women expect men to feel and respond like women. While Martians tend to pull away and silently *think* about what's bothering them, Venusians feel an instinctive need to *talk* about what's bothering them. I had filled that need with Ehris.

One of the hardest lessons in life is letting go. I knew that when we forgive ourselves, we remove the chains from the past and allow ourselves to live freely in the present. To forgive yourself, though, you have to acknowledge you did something wrong, and that was the hardest thing for me to understand. *It wasn't my fault, it wasn't my fault*, I would assure myself. But that little voice would sneak up on me when I least expected it, and whisper, *if you really loved them, you could have fixed them...If you had only tried a little harder, you could have fixed it all....*

There is no such place as Andy Hardy's Carvel, Idaho, where all the endings are happy ones. Although my mother hadn't followed her own advice to walk away from destructive people, I had. My parents forced me to choose between them, and I chose not to choose.

CHAPTER SIXTY

Ehris

Unsuspectingly, I began my herbal studies in the safety of my gardens. Originally, I just wanted to grow vegetables. Then something magical started to happen. As I spent time alone weeding, watering, and working, the plants themselves began to mentor me. When I researched how to harvest the catnip I had planted for Harry, I stumbled upon the use of catnip for menstrual cramps, insomnia, and nightmares. This led to a strong thirst to learn the healing energies of all the plants I was growing. I came home from Woodbury Library with piles of medicinal herb books, and signed up for classes. As nerdy as it may sound, reading about the Latin names of herbs and their actions was cathartic. I loved the idea that every malady has a cousin that heals it.

It wasn't just the actual herbs that cured me. It was also medicinal to work with them. I planted borage, mostly because of the unusual look of the flower; but when I brewed tea from its leaves and blossoms, it lifted my heavyheartedness. In one of my old botanical books, I read that jousters used borage because they believed it brought them courage, which was what it did for me. It gave me the courage to release my anger at Jose and my grandfather, as well as my sadness over the dead end of our Brazilian dream and Nazey's situation. It gave me the courage to know that since I had healed myself, I could help others. I took the advice of one of my dog-eared herb books which included a quote by Maya Angelou, "As soon as healing takes place, go out and heal somebody else."

The way you help heal the world is to start with your own family. My dad had always been open to the natural healing arts. Since I was sure there was a flower essence that could help him, I tried many times to find out exactly what he was feeling. Through my flower essence studies, I knew that there were numerous remedies for an emotion like grief, but also how important it was to be specific, so you knew which one to choose. My dad acted like his heart had been so thoroughly and irreparably broken that there could be no real joy again, but when I tried to pin down his emotional symptoms, he would simply respond, "I'm just tired."

By now, I had my own copy of the 406-page *Flower Essence Repertory*, as well as 96 of the essences. I devoured the book. It was my bedtime reading, Bible, and obsession. I was determined to find the cure for my dad, and pored over every remedy. When I read about Poison Oak, I knew I had found it:

Patterns of imbalance: Fear of intimate contact, protective of personal boundaries; fear of being violated; hostile or distant.

Positive qualities: Emotional openness and vulnerability, ability to be close and make contact with others.

My mom agreed. "Holy smoke! It sounds like that description was written exactly for him! How should we give it to him?"

"I want to see if flower essences *really* work. I think they do, since they worked for us, but since he's so messed up, this will be the real test," I explained. "Can we not tell him he's taking it?"

"I think that's a good idea. It can't hurt him, and if it's the wrong remedy, it won't do anything, right?"

"Yeah. It's pretty weird that actual poison oak can give you a rash, but the flower essence doesn't. But are we being like Nazey with the Librax?" I asked in concern.

"No, I don't think so. Flower essences get at the root of things and fix them. Tranquilizers are just Band-Aids. I don't think he'll ever get better if we don't help him. We can't keep living with this sadness. I say we do it."

That night, I put four drops of Poison Oak flower essence in his iced tea. In the morning, my mom put four drops in his daily shot glass of apple cider vinegar. When he came home from work, he seemed different.

"How you doin', Chaunce-man?" he asked cheerfully, as he knelt to scratch Chauncey's stomach. My mom and I, sitting on the couch, turned our heads in slow motion to stare at each other with raised eyebrows. At dinner, he excitedly told us about his day, then went to the kitchen and emptied the dishwasher.

Still at the table, my mom mouthed animatedly, "Holy cow! Can you believe it?!"

Out of the corner of my mouth, I whispered, "Mommy, do you think it could be working that fast?"

"I don't know," she shrugged hopefully. "Let's see how it goes."

The next day, my dad suggested that the three of us go for a hike at Steep Rock in Washington. Throughout the car ride, he never stopped talking. From the back seat, my mom texted me, "Holy mackerel! What's up with Chatty Cathy?" As we began our hike, stories from my dad's childhood, which I had never heard before, streamed out like the winding river we walked along. My mom lagged behind, and I think she did it on purpose. I heard about a lost goat he chased all over Newtown, and how his former kindergarten teacher spotted him leading it by the horns and gave them both a ride home. I had no idea he'd had a cow named Josephine when he was a little boy, or that his first dog had been named Arfie. He used to buy bubble gum in the morning, then sell it to kids (at a profit) before school started. In first grade, a nun made him stay in for recess for the whole year because he had crammed an entire pink Hostess Sno Ball in his mouth during lunch. And then came the bad stuff.

Possibly for the first time in his life, my dad exposed his vulnerable side as we paused by a maple tree. He told me with tears in his eyes, "I couldn't protect them, Ehris. I let them down. I should have saved my sisters from my son-of-a-bitch brother."

"But Mommy said you were only a baby," I said. "You couldn't have stopped it."

"I didn't know it happened until Mommy and I were already married," my dad began in his usual factual way. "Aunt Jean was going to a psychiatrist for depression. She didn't even know she had repressed memories. When the psychiatrist worked with her, it all came back. She came over to our house and told us what she remembered. She had been five years old when it all happened. She said Wayne used to rape them every Thursday night when our parents went grocery shopping. He always made Mary be the lookout. That night, Mary saw their car pull up the driveway, but didn't say anything. Then my goddamn father beat my sisters and told them it was their fault and the three of them asked for it.

"All Jean wanted was for our parents to apologize for what had happened. I arranged a day when my parents and Jean were going to come over to our house. Jean locked herself in our bathroom because she was afraid to confront them. I finally got her to come out, but my parents refused to admit they were wrong. They said they would handle it the same way all over again. All Jean wanted was an apology. They wouldn't give it to her."

"So that's why you stopped seeing your parents?" I asked.

"I didn't want anything to do with either of them."

I didn't really know what to say, but it seemed like my dad needed absolution. "None of this stuff was your fault. Your brother, your parents, Jose, and Grandpa were all creepy jerks. You've had a lot of junk dumped on you, and you have to stop blaming yourself."

"It *was* my fault, Ehris. It was my idea for us to move to Brazil. I'm the one that became friends with Jose…and that night when Grandpa's esophagus burst, I never should have driven him to the emergency room…I should have just let him stay home like he wanted…he would have died, and Nazey wouldn't be in Laurel Ridge…."

"Stop!" I cut him off. "Nobody blames you! Nobody has *ever* blamed you. We told you a million times before, you didn't drag us to Brazil. We all wanted to go. I have no idea what happened with Jose, and we'll never know. Of course you had to drive Grandpa to the hospital. You never could have known what he would wind up doing. But we're all okay. We survived."

I knew he wouldn't really acknowledge what I'd said, but when he took a deep breath and asked, "How's ice cream sound?" I knew he'd heard me.

As we walked back to the tree stump where my mom was waiting, I thought about a quote I'd read by Angela Blount: "Everybody's damaged. It's just a question of how badly, and whether you're healing or still bleeding."

CHAPTER SIXTY-ONE

Velya

After a long period of sadness, you might see a small bright spot one day, and before you know it, the world will become a lovely place again.

I was unloading the dishwasher one Sunday morning, and from the kitchen window, I could see Jim sitting on a large rock. Something about the way he was sitting caught my attention. It was his shoulders. They weren't limp, but there was a slackness to them. He almost looked relaxed. I pulled on the pair of L.L. Bean boots I always left on the mudroom floor and headed up to the rock. Jim had been spending a lot of time out there, and was wearing one of the brown canvas Carhartt jackets I had come to identify with him. They're durable, made to last, and worn by hard workers. This one had frayed cuffs, and the corduroy collar and pleated elbows were finally wearing out. These jackets were so stiff that when he came into the house for lunch, took them off, and left them on the floor like he always did, they stood up by themselves. The front pockets always contained nails or screws that I overlooked until I heard them clinking around in the dryer.

I leaned over and squeezed his shoulder, which passed for a hug after so many years of marriage. "What the heck are you doing out here? You've got the *I was thinking* face going on." Seeing his face now reminded me that this was the first time he'd looked this way since Brazil. "I think we should build a barn up here," he said. "I found some of the fieldstones from the original foundation."

I was flabbergasted. For years, I had joked and grumbled about Jim's bubbling pots of new ideas. It wasn't until I saw him on the rock in his ratty Carhartt jacket that I realized all his pots had grown stone cold. It wasn't that he was making *wrong* decisions. He wasn't making *any* decisions. He had sewn parts of himself back together, but had used quick, temporary basting stitches. His seams weren't straight. I missed the person he had been when he was in the midst of planning and creating. I missed his projects and dreams. It's the little things, always the little things, that get you in the end and help you see things clearly.

People say you don't know what you've got until it's gone—that you don't realize the true value of something until you no longer have it. The truth was, I knew what I had; I just never thought I'd lose it. Perhaps you must lose everything to be able to appreciate anything. It's very simple, the relativity of suffering. The worst way to miss somebody is when they're right beside you.

I had come very close to losing Jim—not in a divorce sort of way, but there were scattered pieces of him all over the place. He was like one of those connect-the-dots activities for kids in which the picture can't be seen until you draw the lines. It was hard to get used to the sudden absence of such an important person in my life. It reminded me of when I'd stopped teaching after Mic was born and the weird, uneasy feeling I'd gotten, like I was forgetting to do something. If I went out to lunch, I felt guilty, like I was sneaking around. My life until that point had pivoted around some form of a job, and all of a sudden, it was gone.

To someone else, it might have seemed a simple thing, but I knew that in saying he wanted to build a barn, Jim was connecting his dots with our present and sketching the outline of tomorrow. Another woman might have argued that we didn't need a barn. The person I used to be might have argued with him, too. But this wasn't about a barn— it was Jim's way of showing his love for us, for the family. He had tried to do it in Brazil, but in his mind, he had failed. Just as I openly displayed my love for him through my writing, it was my responsibility to accept *his* love as it was offered.

"I'd love to have a barn out here," I said.

He opened the back doors of his work van. It was stacked from bottom to top with lumber and plywood. I don't know how big he was planning on making the barn, but this first load of materials was going to keep him busy for a while.

"How long did you have this cooked up?" I laughed. "You knew exactly what I'd say, didn't you?'

And then he got the look he used to get when I caught him in something. It wasn't sheepish, because that would imply that he was embarrassed. It was more like he was smiling at an inside joke, and I already knew his punchline. I leaned into him and said, "Even when you heal, you're never what you were before. You can't go back. You can't change the past. It just *is*, Jim. It's never going to be the life we had before. But the best revenge is living a happy life."

When we turned to walk to the house, he kept his arm around me and I was aware, as I always was with Jim, of feeling small. Like butterflies in their chrysalises waiting for the perfect moment, out on that rock, we had emerged from the protective cocoons we had spun. Any speck of our caterpillar selves had disappeared. It was impossible to change back into what we had been before Brazil. Healing is like the transformation of becoming a butterfly—it goes through stages. Just like a butterfly, Jim had awakened in his own time. He let go and accepted what was. What seemed to be our world falling apart was actually our world changing, because the world changes when we change.

That night, Jim slowly undressed me in our old iron bed. I had forgotten he had a way of removing my socks, underwear, and jeans in one fell swoop. I had forgotten about the way he used to kiss me. He didn't stop, not even as he unclasped my bra and slowly slid just the sleeves of my T-shirt and sweater from my arms. It felt as if I was naked inside a pillowcase. He pushed the clothing layers into a bunched-up tangle of fabrics around my neck, never taking his lips from mine except for one teasing second when he pulled the clothes over my head, only to instantly kiss me again as if we had been parted for years.

This wasn't the home-from-a-three-day-business-trip sex of our early marriage, when Jim raced into the house and tore off most of my clothes before the dome light had gone out in the car—but it had the same excitement and anticipation as "beginning sex" when you first meet. The unzipping, unfastening, and unbuttoning had a teasing heat. Jim focused on my earlobes, hands, and lower back...those unsung erotic spots. There was none of the hurried kiss, kiss, kiss, tweak,

tweak, tweak the nipple, sex of the past year. Instead, he moved up and down my body like Billy Joel tinkling the ivories, and I had no idea where he was going next. With an exciting newness that was at the same time comfortably familiar, we took a white pebble out of our bucket. When Jim finally entered me, it was as if his body whispered, "I'm back. We're home."

PART FIVE

One does not discover new lands without consenting
to lose sight of the shore for a very long time.

—ANDRÉ GIDE,
The Counterfeiters: A Novel

CHAPTER SIXTY-TWO

Ehris

Nazey's ashes are on the mantle of the home she never wanted to leave. Uncle Jordan told us that my grandfather, who wouldn't bring her home when she was alive, sobbed, "I just can't bear to be apart from her." There was no funeral, memorial service, or closure. The last time I saw her was in the hospital three years earlier, when she told my mom and me about her tragic estrangement from her brother, Chuck.

When Nazey died, my mom became the matriarch of a shrinking family. I'd held a tiny sliver of hope that my grandfather would die first, and Nazey would then be able to live with us and enjoy family dinners, chickens clucking outside her bedroom window, Netflix movies, and poking around in thrift shops. Now, with Mic in Puerto Rico, my grandparents gone, and Uncle Jordan avoiding us for some unexplained reason, it felt lonesome and final. After years of trying to figure out what was going on in the minds of Mic, my dad, Nazey, my grandfather, and Jose, I'd had enough of trying to analyze people. I was still finding my way. I couldn't afford to be thrown off track by examining what was causing Uncle Jordan's distance, and I didn't really care.

A year and a half later, I was reminded that life can change in an instant, and that instant can last forever.

"Oh, my god! Ehris! Come here!" my mom shrieked from the living room.

I was in the kitchen straining an elderflower tincture, and thought, *ugh, she's being so dramatic. I'm sure it's just some stupid thing on Facebook.* Ignoring her, I got out a label for the tincture bottle.

"Ehris! I'm not kidding! Come here!" she insisted.

Annoyed, I finished what I was doing, and plopped beside her on the couch. She kept wildly pointing at her laptop screen. "Oh, my god! Oh, my god! Look!"

"What?" I sighed, with attitude.

"I got a Facebook message from some guy named Chuck Ehrismann."

"Wait. What? Nazey's brother? Isn't he dead?" I asked, confused.

"I think it's his kid!"

"He had a *kid*?" I asked.

"Read this!" my mom demanded, handing me her laptop. Scrolling through the message, I read:

Hello, my name is Charles A. Ehrismann. My father was Charles A. Ehrismann, Jr., son of Charles A. Ehrismann and Ann (McWilliams) Ehrismann. My dad was Neysa Ehrismann Jancz's brother.

I really don't even know how to begin this conversation. My dad and mother separated when I was a baby in New Jersey. I only know of him through some old photographs and stories. I always knew that he had an older sister, but I didn't know her name.

For about the last 30 years or so, I have been searching for family. It's Christmas Eve. Today in my office, for some reason, I decided to search again. I decided that after this last try, I would stop searching and move on with my life. Today, when I typed in my grandparents' names, I discovered Neysa's obituary…I am sorry for her passing.

A little bit about me:

I was born in New Jersey on January 27, 1968 at the Margaret Hague Hospital in Jersey City, but after my mother and father separated, my mother moved to South America for a few years to run her textiles business. I returned to South Florida, where I grew up and began a beautiful family. My wife, Danielle, and I are now living in Portland, Oregon, on the Columbia River with our two kids.

Velya…I'm a little overwhelmed, and really don't know how to approach this. But it would be an absolute pleasure and honor if we could talk. I am wondering if you would consider a conversation, or, at the very least, Facebook or e-mail messages. I would love for you to see my family pictures. Danielle is more active on Facebook, so I would look her up. I would love to talk.

Sincerely,
Charles "Chuck" Albert Ehrismann

Then I read my mom's first response:

What!!?? We're relatives?! Wait a sec, I have to go back and read your message…

First cousins!

I am in shock!!! If you knew how many times I searched for Chuck (my mom's brother) online, you would faint. I don't even know where to start! Our daughter's first name is Ehris.

I saw that. Sorry to shock you. I've spent years looking for my family.

It's a good shock. I have a cousin?! I have a relative?!

For 40 years, Chuck had stared at a black and white photo, given to him by his mother, of a stunning unknown woman sitting on a boulder. The only clue was *1949 Keansburg, New Jersey* penciled on the back, but Chuck suspected she was family and held the key to his own identity. He emailed us the photo and asked, *Do you know who this woman is?*

That's my mother! my mom typed excitedly in response. *I've never seen that photo!*

Over the course of his search to find his father, Chuck learned that he had died in 1990. Chuck had searched every possible woman's name he could think of in order to find his dad's older sister. With names like Neysa, Velya, and Ehris, he didn't have a chance of finding us—until the obituary, which included the names of Neysa's parents.

Chuck, Danielle, Essie, and Aidan's visit that summer was the final piece of healing for all of us. Chuck found out who he was. My dad's cracked protective shell fell away when he talked about Nazey's wacky side with tenderness. My mom was able to allow the good memories of Nazey to filter through as she shared family stories with Chuck. I made peace with the past through this new beginning.

The hours we spent crying and laughing outside in the Adirondack chairs were magical. At one point, my mom disappeared and came back with the black velvet jewelry box.

"I thought you might like to have this," my mom said, handing Chuck the box. "Your dad bought it in Italy when he was in the navy, and gave it to my mother. There was a second one, but she had me give it to Jordan."

"A cameo?" Chuck asked, fingering the only tangible piece of his father.

My mom said with tears in her eyes, "Even when I was a little kid, and didn't know the story about their estrangement, I liked thinking about the fact that he actually picked it out especially for his sister, that he touched it, and carried it safely home to her in his pocket."

"Before you appeared, it was too painful for any of us to look at it," I explained.

"No, no, I can't take it," Chuck protested, closing the box and handing it to me. "It was meant for your grandmother. Don't you see the significance of the cameo, Ehris? The three women on it represent you, your mom, and your grandmother."

I gasped. Until that moment, I had only allowed myself to think of the Nazey who was addicted to narcotics and tolerant of abuse. The one who took advantage of my mom's talent for dealing with problem people, dumped everything on her, and turned her into the family social worker. When I saw the three goddesses on the cameo, I realized that I never knew the real Nazey. I think I saw a glimpse of her when I was five years old, when we curled up together on my bunk bed and sang the entire *Phantom of the Opera* soundtrack. I felt grown-up, and she radiated the abandon of a little girl. It was the only time I can remember her not being on guard.

A grounded female has the potential to be a complete circle. Within her is the power to create, nurture, and transform. In Celtic cultures, maidens were seen as flowers, mothers were the fruit, and elder women were the seeds. The seeds held the knowledge, potential, and power of all the other archetypes. Nazey had been wise in some ways, but she hadn't been nourished enough as a maiden to ever become a seed.

"Ehris, don't you see that you're a healer?" Chuck continued. "It's your wounds that enable you to be compassionate with the wounds of others. You've turned every tear into a pearl of wisdom. The cameo should be your reminder of that."

Chuck eased the pain of the past, my dad saved us monetarily, and my mom was the lifeline that sewed our family back together. She said we'd all become better versions of ourselves.

When women who need healing are mended, they should spread the word, hold out their hands, and share some love and laughter with a new member of the sisterhood who needs help. If I turn into my mom, or even half the woman she is, I'll consider my life a successful one. Every daughter deserves a mother, and every mother deserves a daughter, who'll listen, take her side, and tell the truth (or not, depending on what she needs). A woman you can count on, no matter what.

For my 24th birthday that year, I didn't get a Vitamix or a dehydrator. Together, my parents and I went to a jewelry store, and I picked out a 14-karat gold setting for the cameo. Wearing it around my neck is like wearing an amulet. It's my connection to the past, but it's also my reminder that I have survived my deepest wounds. The wreckage I overcame has left me stronger and more resilient. What hurt me has actually made me better able to face the present. Wounding and healing aren't opposites. They're part of the same thing.

CHAPTER SIXTY-THREE

Ehris

Life's too short to live in fear. That pull you feel, nagging at you every day, is real. Your path probably won't make sense to your family or friends. People will weigh in with comments like, "Won't you miss speaking English?"

"Don't they have those candiru fish there that swim up into a man's penis, then eat it from the inside?"

"What about your 401ks?"

We were visiting Mic in Puerto Rico for Thanksgiving. It was the first family vacation we'd taken in seven years, since coming back from Brazil. Sitting by the pool at the Casa Grande Mountain Retreat in Caonillas, we felt excitement and hysteria bubble up in us like Diet Coke and Mentos about to explode out of a soda bottle. It was the same feeling we'd experienced on Jose and Isabela's laundry room floor, when our dream to open the *hotel fazenda* had ignited.

"I had no idea the mountains of Puerto Rico were so beautiful!" my mom exclaimed. "And the temperature's so much nicer here than in San Juan!"

"Mommy, I've been telling you this ever since I moved here!" Mic admonished.

"This view looks like something from *Gorillas in the Mist*," my dad said in admiration.

I flipped through the tropical herbalism book I had bought in the gift shop and added, "Wow! Did you know that clove, arnica, and almonds grows here? That's so cool!"

"This is what I've been trying to tell you guys," Mic said in exasperation. "Puerto Rico is like the best parts of the U.S. and the best parts of Brazil. You guys never got to live your dream. You could do it here!"

"Mic, we were too messed up to even think about it before," my mom responded.

"You know what would be *so* cool?" Mic said excitedly. "If we bought an old *hacienda* here and made it into an eco-tourism destination!"

"Yeah! Can we have horses?" I asked.

"Duh, Ehris." Mic sighed.

"Ehris, did you see the cacao trees at the coffee plantation tour this morning?" my dad asked. "We could make our own chocolate!"

"You know, I always thought I'd be excellent at running a bed and breakfast," my mom mused. "Mic, how old are these haciendas? Could we find a cool, old one?"

"There aren't a lot of old ones left because of the termites, but I bet we could find one! Should I see if I can find any online?" Mic asked, reaching for his phone.

"Maybe we could find one that could be a working farm *and* a tourist place," my dad said.

"We need the perfect name for it," I ruminated.

"Don't worry," said my mom. "It'll come to us."

"Yo! You guys! Listen!" Mic announced. "This is the first one that came up. It's an old coffee plantation with 97 acres.

It says it's from 1860, and they grow coffee, plantains, lemons, and oranges."

"Are there any pictures?" I asked.

Within minutes, Mic, speaking Spanish, had called the realtor and arranged for us to see the hacienda the next day—our last day in Puerto Rico.

The winding drive through the mountains gave me time to think about my family. What had happened hadn't destroyed us, either individually or as a whole. If people knew what we were now considering, I was sure many would criticize: "You're taking too big a chance. Did you learn nothing from Brazil?" Hopefully, others would applaud: "Good for you. You're following your bliss."

I loved my family. We had met defeat, but we were willing to try again. And if it turned out to be a mistake…so what?

The realtor met us at the top of the hacienda's long palm-lined driveway. Before I even got out of the car, I saw myself carrying a wicker basket of lemons up to the second-story veranda of *The Lemon House*.

ℰ∂

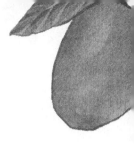

ACKNOWLEDGMENTS

❧

In August 1914, the British Imperial Trans-Antarctic Expedition, under the leadership of Ernest Shackleton, left England with the goal of crossing Antarctica via the South Pole. Their ship, *Endurance*, became trapped in ice, then drifted for 10 months, was crushed in pack ice, and sank. The 28 crewmembers then drifted on ice floes for another five months. They finally escaped in *Endurance*'s three lifeboats to Elephant Island, where they survived on seal meat, penguins, and their dogs. Shackleton and five men sailed 800 miles in a 20 foot whale boat—a 16-day journey across a stretch of dangerous ocean—before landing on the southern side of South Georgia Island. In the final push, Shackleton, Frank Worsley, and Tom Crean—roped together, with screws in their boots for traction—traveled continuously for 36 hours before reaching Stromness, a whaling station. Before they walked into Stromness, covered in blubber smoke and unrecognizable, Shackleton quoted the Canadian poet Robert Service, ". . . we had grown bigger in the bigness of the whole." Four months later, after attempting four separate relief expeditions, Shackleton succeeded in rescuing his crew from Elephant Island. Not one of Shackleton's crew had died.

Shackleton's men remained in relatively good spirits throughout the entire ordeal. His "secret" had nothing to do with choosing polar explorers or seasoned wilderness guys—he very carefully chose men who were cheerful and optimistic (along with being good at their professions). His leadership style is now studied by "leaders" all over the world.

Like Shackleton and his crew, we braved the unknown, discovered something greater than ourselves, and became better people for appreciating it. We were grounded, lost almost everything, and became better versions of ourselves. We have "grown bigger in the bigness of the whole."

We're grateful to a varied cast of characters who helped see this book to fruition.

Jo Heck encouraged us to enter a Facebook contest sponsored by When Words Count Retreat in Rochester, Vermont. When we won a four-night stay, we planned to hunker down and work on new class ideas. We had no intention of writing a book—but it happened.

It's important that authors and publishers are right for each other. When we told Dede Cummings that we had received a blurb from Dr. Christiane Northrup and she audibly gasped, we knew she and Green Writers Press were the right fit for us!

Our first editor, Peg Moran, put an encouraging spin on our manuscript edits. We miss her 3:00 A.M. emails with gentle nudges like, "I know you toned down the ickiness factor, but it's still pretty strong and in the book a lot. I understand Velya's interest in the way things work, but most readers aren't going to share your interest to that extent…"

Asha Hossain agreed to take a second look at a cover idea slated for the junk pile, and turned it into the vibrant cover it is today.

One can never have too many librarian friends. Ours are not only champions of books; they've supported us from the outset. Thank you to Marla Martin, Sue Piel, Suzanne Garvey, and Ann Szaley.

When we call Marilyn Atlas "a character," that's about the highest compliment we can bestow upon a person. She helped us see that by opening with the betrayal, we weren't giving away our story.

There aren't many photographers who would willingly agree to a photoshoot with a Buff Orpington chicken (or any chicken, for that matter). Even though we broke one of her lights and her backdrop was pooped on by Little Joanie Pekar (the chicken), Lora Karam has become a good friend.

Aureliano Oliveira helped us navigate our abbreviated Brazilian adventure.

Thank you to Samantha Figueira Rafoss, who helped make one of us fluent in Portuguese. A teacher by chance, a friend by choice…

Our hawk-eyed editor, Cathryn Lykes, fixed those pesky manuscript issues: potbelly pig vs. potbellied pig, that vs. which, and paint pony vs. painted pony. One of her suggestions prompted a lively firehouse/fire department/fire station Facebook debate.

Since this book's conclusion, we've gone on to create *Grounded Goodwife* (groundedgoodwife.com). The encouragement of our "charter members" has brought us to where we are today.

We spent many, many writing and editing hours at New Morning Market and Ayla's Bagel & Deli in Woodbury, CT. Thanks for the moral support and free samples!

When someone you've idolized for years on PBS blurbs your book, it's pretty understandable that when you open the envelope containing the blurb, your screams can be heard three states away. Thank you to Dr. Christiane Northrup, author of *Mother-Daughter Wisdom.*

Our weekly acupuncture sessions with Andrea Coakley started as grief therapy, but blossomed into a friendship we both cherish above all others.

And finally, to Jose. You dynamited our "breathtaking piece of folly," but you didn't exterminate our resilient spirit. Thanks for showing us how strong we really are.

WORKS CONSULTED

❧

Barrett, Tracy. *Growing Up in Colonial America*. Brookfield, CT: Millbrook, 1995. Print.

Berkin, Carol. *First Generations: Women in Colonial America*. New York: Hill and Wang, 1996. Print.

Carmack, Sharon DeBartolo. *Your Guide to Cemetery Research*. Cincinnati, OH: Betterway, 2002. Print.

Earle, Alice Morse. *Home-Life in Colonial Days*. New York: MacMillan, 1899. Print.

Finley, Harry. "What Did American and European Women Use for Menstruation in the Past?"

What Did Women DO? 1 Jan. 1999. Web. 20 Oct. 2014.

Hawke, David Freeman. *Everyday Life in Early America*. New York: Harper & Row, 1988. Print.

Kaminski, Patricia, and Richard Katz. *Flower Essence Repertory: a Comprehensive Guide to North American and English Flower Essences for Emotional and Spiritual Well-Being*. Flower Essence Society, 2004.

Perl, Lila. *Slumps, Grunts, and Snickerdoodles.* New York: Seabury, 1975. Print.

Tannenbaum, Rebecca J. *Health and Wellness in Colonial America.* Santa Barbara, CA: Greenwood, 2012. Print.

The Old Herb Doctor: His Secrets and Treatments. [New ed. North Hollywood, CA: Newcastle Pub., 1981]. Print.

Tannenbaum, Rebecca. *The Healer's Calling: Women and Medicine in Early New England.* Ithaca: Cornell UP, 2002. Print.

Taylor, Dale. *The Writer's Guide to Everyday Life in Colonial America.* Cincinnati, OH: Writer's Digest, 1997. Print.

Tunis, Edwin. *Colonial Living.* New York: Thomas Y. Crowell, 1957. Print.

Ulrich, Laurel Thatcher. *A Midwife's Tale: The Life of Martha Ballard, Based on Her Diary, 1785-1812.* New York: Knopf, 1990. Print.

Ulrich, Laurel Thatcher. *Good Wives: Image and Reality in the Lives of Women in Northern New England, 1650-1750.* New York, NY: Knopf, 1982. Print.

Volo, James M., and Dorothy Denneen Volo. *Daily Life on the Old Colonial Frontier.* Westport, CT: Greenwood, 2002. Print.

Warner, J. F. *Colonial American Home Life.* New York: F. Watts, 1993. Print.

Warwick, Edward. *Early American Dress: The Colonial and Revolutionary Periods.* New York: Bonanza, 1965. Print.

Wertz, Richard W., and Dorothy C. Wertz. *Lying-In: A History of Childbirth in America.* New York: Free, 1977. Print.

MEET EHRIS AND VELYA

❧

Ehris Urban, owner of Woodbury, CT's *Grounded Holistic Wellness*, believes, "if you're grounded, you can navigate even the bumpiest roads in peace." She grew up in a family passionate about holistic medicine. Ehris is a certified herbalist and holistic nutritionist, and a graduate of the New England School of Homeopathy. Additionally, Ehris is a Flower Essence Therapy practitioner. She became interested in Reiki as a teenager and attained Reiki Master certification at age 17. Ehris is also a certified Ingham Method reflexologist. A graduate of Western Connecticut State University with a B.A. in Anthropology/Sociology, she is also a certified ESL teacher. Ehris enjoys beekeeping, tending her organic vegetable and herb gardens, and working in her apothecary.

Velya Jancz-Urban lives her life by the adage, "there is no growth without change." Zany and gregarious, she is a teacher, author, former Brazilian dairy farm owner, and expert on herstory unsanitized. Moving into a 1770 Connecticut farmhouse ignited Velya's obsession with the colonial era, and led to her entertainingly-informative presentation, *The Not-So-Good Life of the Colonial Goodwife*, followed by *The Not-So Golden Life of the Gilded Age Wife*. She has been married for 36 years and is the mother of two grown children. Velya has a few too many rescue dogs and cats, is happiest with a fresh stack of library books, loves thrift shops, and is passionate about alternative medicine.

As *Grounded Goodwife* (groundedgoodwife.com), the funny and frank duo believe in taking inner responsibility for one's wellness, and share their "recipe" for wholeness through hands-on holistic workshops and "gal power" presentations.